What's Next

Striving for happiness after heartbreaking loss

by

Robert Buren

© 2021 Robert Buren. All rights reserved. No part of this publication may be reproduced, distributed, or transmitted in any form or by any means, including photocopying, recording, or other electronic or mechanical methods, without prior written permission of the author, except in case of brief quotations in critical reviews and certain other non-commercial uses permitted by copyright law.

Published by No Better Time Inc.

eBook Edition ISBN: 978-1-7779186-1-3

Paperback Edition ISBN: 978-1-7779186-0-6

Photo Credits:
Front Cover: FinisherPix®
Back Cover: Sabrina Haque
Profile Photo: Niall Pinder

Dedication

For my daughters Chloe and Zara.

Preface

Before We Begin

What makes a story worth telling? I've asked that question countless times as I've written down my thoughts, feelings, and experiences from the past 13 years. I think the answer is there's comfort and inspiration in knowing that you're not alone. The specifics of my journey are unique, but we're all travelling roads that present unexpected hardships, and it's up to each of us to decide if we're going to stay the course, find a detour, take a rest, or call for help. When you see parallels between your life and choices and those of another, you get a broader perspective on your own challenges and perhaps some motivation to act. I share my story of having navigated the challenges in my life, hoping it will help you do the same in yours.

But before you start reading about my life, write about yours and jot down responses to these two questions:

What's the worst thing in life that could possibly happen to you?

What's the hardest thing in life that you're dealing with currently?

We'll come back to these questions.

Table of Contents

Introduction – Achieving the Impossible v

Chapter 1 – The Good Life 1

Chapter 2 – One Day in the Woods 11

Chapter 3 – Doctors and Hospitals 22

Chapter 4 – This Guy Can Fly 36

Chapter 5 – Family, Friends & Strangers 53

Chapter 6 – Pushing Hard – Going Nowhere 68

Chapter 7 – Training in All its Forms 85

Chapter 8 – The Cruelest Pain 111

Chapter 9 – The Road to Kona 125

Chapter 10 – The Ironman World Championships 153

Chapter 11 – Lessons Learned 170

Chapter 12 – Not Again 176

Chapter 13 – Today 184

Acknowledgements 186

Introduction

Achieving the Impossible

As the sun rises and reveals what seems to be a perfect day, I'm thrilled. I'm far from my home in Canada; it's October 8th, 2016, 6:45 AM, and I've already been awake for hours. I'm treading water in Hawaii's Kailua Bay, surrounded by 2,300 of the world's fastest triathletes. As helicopters thump overhead, we wait for the cannon to fire to start this world-renowned endurance race.

There's a crowd along the water's edge that buzzes with excitement and feeds off the energy from the eager, determined athletes. The spectators are triathlon crazed enthusiasts, family, and friends, drawn from all over the world for the championship event. The whole island has been taken over by triathletes and their fans, assembled for what is known to the triathlete community as the "Big Dance."

Every athlete knows that this is their chance to do something extraordinary. Not everyone is going to make it to the end, but all of us are going to push ourselves to the peak of our physical and mental capacities. Today is the Ironman World Championships.

The "Ironman" is a 226 km (140.6 miles) long-distance triathlon race with a seventeen-hour time limit. The first stage is 3.8 kilometres (km) of swimming, followed by 180 km of cycling, and concluded by a full 42.2 km marathon. Around the world, there are typically 25 Ironman races each year, with over 50,000 athletes racing to test themselves. Only the best (less than 2,400) will qualify for a spot at the World Championships in Hawaii each year, and at that race in October, more than 100 athletes that start the race won't be able to finish. For those who can, the average competitor will lose about four percent of their body weight by the time they reach the finish line. For many reasons, it's known as one of the world's toughest endurance races.

I'm excited to be here with the other competitors, only I'll be attempting the race a little differently than most. I won't be using my legs. When I cross that finish line—*if* I cross that finish line—I'm going to be doing it in a wheelchair.

I'm nervous—everyone is nervous—but I want to be here. Badly. Most able-bodied people think an Ironman is impossible, especially competing in one with just their arms. But I think it is possible. Here I am, determined to be the first Canadian with paraplegia to ever complete this epic event. Failure is not an option.

In 2009, as I recovered from a life-altering accident, I watched the Ironman World Championships on TV and marvelled at a kid from California whom the TV crew followed throughout the race. He had broken his back in a dirt biking accident a couple of years earlier, resulting in paraplegia. I wondered if I had it in me. Could I be strong enough one day? Could I take the suffering and not give up? In the back of my mind, I had this belief that if I could do this race, then I could do anything. No one could call me disabled. I'd still be able to make myself and my girls proud.

In 2008, I was living a blessed life. I had an amazing family and a rewarding career, enjoying all my passions (most of which included two wheels). I had my life planned out and was executing it beautifully. I was in control, right up until the moment I wasn't. In an instant, I found myself paralyzed from the chest down in an accident. Everything changed.

This book is not about what happens when life throws a wrench in your plans. It's about life taking a crowbar and breaking your back with it. It's about an active 37-year-old, married with two daughters, suddenly having to figure out what the fuck just happened and how the hell he is going to fix things for himself and those around him. It's about striving to overcome the challenges that a disability, the world, and most importantly, your own expectations present to you on the road to recovery. And this book is about trying to accept that we are the reader, not the author, of our own story. Ultimately, we must look over the things that happen in our life and try to understand why. Even if we can't. Even when the plot twists in excruciating directions.

My accident was the result of an impulsive decision combined with a lot of bad luck. But that's all it takes to turn a mountain bike ride into a bitch of a life lesson. Lying on the forest floor, from the first moment I realized I couldn't feel my legs, I was already trying to solve the problems this new situation presented me.

Not being able to walk because of my spinal cord injury is only one consequence of my injury. It's the part that everyone sees and might empathize with, but it's actually one of the challenges that I can typically work around. My bigger challenge is something that no one can see: neuropathic pain. Daily, in varying degrees, my skin from my injury on down feels like it's on fire. There's no rhyme or reason, and some days I swear that it even changes with the weather.

For someone who grew up wanting control and predictability, a spinal cord injury messes with your head. The game just changed, and there's no choice but to adapt. I needed a whole new plan to live without the use of my lower body. And I have an unwanted companion called neuropathic pain that pulls me backwards and tries to convince me to give up.

I like a challenge. And I like to work hard. But this was going to be a whole other level of difficult. One thing I knew for certain was that I would have the support of exceptional family and friends, and they would help me overcome any challenge or meet any goal that I set for myself.

The most important thing this experience confirmed for me is that attitude and perspective are everything. Before the accident, I thought I had the game of life figured out. I knew the rules of the game and what I had to do to win. If only it were that simple. Life is much more unpredictable and complicated than I want it to be. You can't anticipate what it's likely to throw your way, and you certainly do not have the control you think. The world does what it wants, and the best you can do is control your own attitude and perspective—the stories you tell yourself. These are the most important things you can control if you want to live a good life, regardless of the challenges that you'll face.

I know that no life is perfect. We all have ups and downs, and I consider myself very lucky to have accomplished some amazing things that I'm proud to share with the wider world. But I've also had my share of dark days that I've suffered in silence. The darkest and most depressing of which were brought about by the side effects of the medications I was prescribed for my pain. Meds that were supposed to ease my burning neuropathic pain symptoms also allowed my brain to contemplate suicide. When your own thoughts scare you, you need to dig deep to push them back.

Not long after my accident, I read a quote that resonated with me: "The greatest pleasure in life is doing what people say you cannot do." I love it, and I took it on as my mantra to motivate my recovery. If you don't think I can do something that I've said I was going to do, then screw you. I'm going to do it anyway. I'm going to do everything I did before my accident and more. I'm going to be a paratriathlete. Just watch me. And if you tell me I can't, I'll now have even more motivation to do it, while having the bonus of proving you wrong.

The Ironman started out as this crazy idea in the back of my head. Most able-bodied people can't imagine doing one part of this race, nevertheless all three disciplines. But that's other people. What about me? The questions bounced around in my head. Could I do it with just my arms? And what for? It's not unheard of for athletes to not finish an Ironman, even after all the work that is required to get to the start line. It's not uncommon for athletes to be pulled from the course for missing a cut-off time. Racers faint, throw up, and even shit themselves. So, do I really want to commit to a sport where I could easily end up in the hospital again? Do I really want to devote so much time and money to something so hard?

The Ironman is frigging tough. It's messed up. But that's why it's the perfect challenge for me. This is the right level of crazy that will get me out of bed in the morning. A goal that will redefine my limits and continuously test my mettle. Yes, all those bad things can happen. But the more I have trained and accomplished, the more I have believed it's a goal I can accomplish.

That's how I find myself here, treading water in Kona Harbor with hundreds of other crazies. I'm just one of them getting ready to do the same course, on the same day, with the same time cut-offs. The only difference is I'm going to do it all with just my arms.

The cannon fires! Can I achieve the impossible?

Chapter 1

The Good Life

As the final minutes of 2007 ticked by, Sabrina and I sat in bed waiting for the ball to drop. As we watched Times Square on TV, we made a list of things we wanted to do in the coming year. I wouldn't call these resolutions, as the purpose wasn't to try and break any bad habits. Rather, it was more a list of goals that we could work towards with confidence that if we achieved them, we'd have the best year of our lives.

Married for eleven years, I've always considered myself to be lucky when it comes to love. I found the girl of my dreams at university when I was only 21. We met in a musical on campus and were married two years later. Sabrina is the perfect girl for me. A kind heart, an infectious smile and laugh, a love of music, and confidence and ability to do anything, while the clichés of calling Sabrina my soul mate or best friend do apply, I prefer "partner" or "buddy." The best word to describe her is "beautiful." Our love is deep and rich, and our support for one another unquestionable.

We tried to live each day being positive and optimistic; we knew how lucky we were—life was great. Sure, it was busy. But that was to be expected with two daughters under five and trying to get ahead. As the girls were getting older, independent and adventurous, we had started to hit our stride. In other words, 2008 had the potential to be exceptional, and this list would help to make it unforgettable.

Looking back, our fondest memories of the previous year involved being active outside. With a new 21-foot camping trailer, we had explored provincial parks throughout Ontario. Our favourite campgrounds all had beaches, giving us glorious days of sand and water. Late afternoon, we'd pack our beach gear into a little wagon and head back to our campsite for dinner, a shower, story-time by the campfire, and then off to bed. Sharing our love of the outdoors with our little girls made Sabrina and me happy. Camping was something we wanted more of in 2008—it definitely made the list.

When we weren't camping or doing other family activities, Sabrina and I had our own, separate passions. Before having Chloe in 2003 and Zara in 2006, if we weren't working, you'd likely find Sabrina riding her horse and me, my motorcycles. With the arrival of our daughters, Sabrina had less free time to spend at the barn, but that was something we'd try to change in 2008. I, however, had the advantage of being able to ride my motorbike throughout the year. With my good friends, we'd organize a few track days each season, and the occasional work trip to sunny U.S. states involved the occasional sport-bike rental where we'd skip out of the conference and find the best roads the location had to offer. My calls home to Sabrina at the end of those days were always a little awkward, as I hesitated sharing too many details of getting out to ride and eating in nice restaurants when she was home alone with two little ones. But for the most part, she was happy for me. In the New Year, I wanted to add even more motorcycling adventures to the list. I played hard because I worked hard.

In the fall of 2007, I finally landed a job with Microsoft Canada. I say finally because it took many years of applying, strategizing, and proving myself at a Microsoft Partner business before I landed my opportunity. After seven interviews with Microsoft during the summer, I started in October as Canada's Partner Capacity Manager. My role was to make sure Canada had enough partners and that those partners had the right skill sets to get software sold, deployed, and utilized. I was finally working with a corporation of Type A personalities. I found a workplace where the expectations were high, and I loved it.

Lastly, one of the big goals that made the list was to finish a half-marathon. Sabrina and I had done 5Ks and 10Ks before, and we liked the challenge of pushing ourselves to do something harder. A half-marathon is 21.2 kilometres, so it's a significant distance to train and complete. Best of all, it was something we would do together.

As the clock struck midnight, we were starting the year empowered with a thoughtful list of goals to work towards. We turned off the lights, kissed, and started our best year yet.

Spring came quickly, and with it, the purchase of a Chariot running stroller for the girls to ride in. This allowed Sabrina and I to train together and have the girls with us. Before having the running stroller, one of us had to stay behind. Sabrina would pack everything the girls could possibly need for a one-hour stroller ride. Beyond the typical things, like a bottle of water and snacks, she had *The Backyardigans* DVD ready to go in the portable player. And, if they started to get cranky after their nap (they always fell asleep for part of the run), we'd tell them where in the stroller they could find the hidden lollipops. That gave us just enough time to get home before they really got out of sorts and demanded to be freed.

For our summer holiday of 2008, we enjoyed a prime camping spot near the beach in Killbear Provincial Park on Georgian Bay. We discovered this site the summer before, and this gem of a campground had everything we loved: soft sandy beaches, running and cycling paths, and a trail up and over large rocks to a scenic lighthouse—all nestled in the beautiful terrain of the Canadian Shield. We pitched a large blue tarp between four trees over the main part of our site, with a dining tent next to our trailer and awning. Turning a basic camping site into a wonderfully comfortable home in the forest for two full weeks was something I took great pride in doing for my girls. I'd climb trees, move dirt, reposition things as many times as needed to get it simply perfect. My dad used to do this for us when I was growing up, and I looked forward to passing those memories and skills down to Chloe and Zara.

As summer came to an end, I was thrilled that I got away for two consecutive track days with my buddies. On Monday, we hosted our regular TGIM (Thank God It's Monday) track day at Shannonville Raceway, and then we headed up to a friend's cottage for a feast and a good night's sleep. The next day we drove a racetrack further north for another epic outing of speed.

There are few things I enjoy more than the smell of burning fuel and rubber, combined with the scream of an engine bouncing off the rev limiter as you hit over 250 km/h. It's perfection to me. I love motorcycling. Like most track days between sessions, on that afternoon, we shared our most thrilling moments of the last outing and then checked our phones to ensure things at home and back at the office were fine. To my surprise, I received an email that announced the winners of Microsoft Canada's performance awards, and I was on the list. Sweet!

My first few months at Microsoft had been a blur of activity. "Microsofties" often refer to this stage as "drinking from the fire hose." Flying around the country, I was meeting with partners, doing data analysis, and strategizing ways to make everything more efficient. The job was going well for me, and within eight months, I had completed some innovative work and shined a light on some new elements of the business that hadn't been looked at before.

One of the things that really excited me about Microsoft was the opportunity to work for a global corporation with offices around the world. I admired my friends and colleagues from Canada that had moved to Redmond, in Washington State, to work at the head office. Some even ventured to work in Asia and Europe. When Sabrina was growing up, her father worked for and actually opened the first Scotiabank branch in India. Then, they lived in Malaysia, where Sabrina completed high school. I was born and raised in London, Ontario—a smaller and conservative city two hours west of Toronto. Even though we'd been living in and around Toronto for the last ten years, admittedly, my world was pretty small. The thought of working and living in foreign countries excited me, and I loved the idea of giving my children diverse and enriching experiences. I was confident that in time, I'd make this happen.

I worked my ass off at Microsoft, and my hard work was recognized. Receiving the President's Award for Outstanding Achievement within a year of being there felt great, and it even included a trip to Hawaii in November 2008 with Sabrina.

In addition to my day job, in 2007, I started a side business with two friends. It was an IT security conference that would run each fall. Leading the creation of a successful business was something that I always wanted to do, and being able to do it with a couple of good friends was a bonus. Even though I had little extra time in my life, I was excited to make this business happen and was confident it would be a success.

Throughout the year, Sabrina accomplished many things on her list, too, one of the more exciting goals being a dressage competition that our girls, her mom, and I were able to attend to cheer her on. If you're not familiar with dressage, I would describe it as ballet for horse and rider.

Sabrina's love for horses began at the age of 11 when she lived in India. She recalls the first few rides being basic and busy, but she was riding and enjoying everything about it. Two years later, in Malaysia, her riding progressed to the next level with better access to quality horses and coaching. When we met in university, she was a member of the equestrian club and found the occasional opportunity to ride and take a lesson. Early in our marriage, before having Chloe and Zara, I saved up for and purchased motorcycles. Sabrina saved and purchased a 3-year-old gelding named Pikasso.

Dressage was her passion, and she pursued it with patience and determination. It requires a unique skill set that is undeniably impressive. The complexity of the movement is directed through subtle communication between horse and rider. Adding to the challenge is the reality that horses can be temperamental, and when the horse decides it wants you off, you're off.

I remember Sabrina's first dressage test quite vividly. She looked beautiful atop her horse, Pikasso, and began executing all of the movements seamlessly. Turning a 20-metre circle to the right, as she approached the centre of the ring, she asked Pikasso to begin cantering. He didn't pick up the canter right away, so she tapped him with her crop to wake him up. Maybe it was the excitement of so many people watching, or maybe he was just being an ass, but he didn't like the crop and began a series of wild bucks. Sabrina held her seat for the first couple, but after the third or fourth buck, she went flying through the air and slammed into the ground.

We all gasped. Chloe and Zara, just four and two years old, looked on with amazement and concern. I stayed with the girls while her coach and support staff ran to her side. After a few minutes, Sabrina walked over to where we were on the grass, and we dusted the sand off of her riding jacket. She was understandably shaken up, and you could see she was holding back tears. There was also a small amount of blood beginning to seep through one of her white gloves. Not one to wallow, Sabrina collected herself and consulted with her coach, who had caught her horse. She had entered two classes, and to the surprise of everyone (except her and me), she was not going to end the day being thrown off her horse. After just a few minutes of rest, Sabrina made her way over to the warmup ring to get back on for her second class. Composed and communicating better with her horse, her second class went much better, and she and Pikasso won a first-place ribbon.

No one would have faulted Sabrina for calling it a day after being thrown off. But the opportunity to excel presented itself—to literally get back on her horse—and she seized the opportunity with the best possible outcome. It was a great lesson for our girls, showing them that you don't call it a day until you've completed what you set out to do.

The next morning Sabrina was stiff and sore. She didn't think Pikasso stepped on her, but she did fall from a considerable height with considerable force. At the chiropractor, she was told to go for x-rays and to not run the half-marathon the next weekend that we'd been training for all year. Knowing my wife as I did and that the race was still five days away, I wasn't surprised that she was determined to do it. Sabrina has always been tough and determined, and when she puts her mind to something, she follows through.

Race morning arrived quickly. Sabrina somewhat gingerly rolled out of bed, popped a couple of Advil and put on her running gear. Her mom came to watch the girls for us, and after eating a small breakfast and filling our water bottles, we headed out the door for our big race.

At 21.1 kilometres, or 13.1 miles, the half-marathon was much more than just a running event to Sabrina and me. It was a milestone-think-big goal that we set for ourselves on New Year's Eve and something that we planned, trained, and suffered for. Getting to the start line was the culmination of eight months of training and shorter races. We were ready to test ourselves, and we were pumped.

As the announcer began to count down to the start, Sabrina and I kissed each other, wished one another good luck, and started our watches. Go! My legs are a lot longer than hers, and I immediately pulled away. I quickly found my groove and felt strong. For the first ten kilometres, I pushed reasonably hard. My heart rate was in the 160s, which I was confident I could maintain without blowing myself up. I crossed the midway point in just under an hour. Cresting the long hill climb, I squeezed a power gel into my mouth, washed it down with a cup of water from the aid station, and tried to increase my pace slightly. Within a few minutes, I caught up with a couple of friends. They were looking good, and I knew they were strong runners, so I hung with them for the next eight or nine kilometres.

With only a couple of kilometres left, I wanted to see how fast I could go. I put my head down, gently pulled away from those maintaining pace, and finished a minute or two ahead of my friends. It was the longest distance I'd ever run in my life, and I did it with a finishing time of one hour and fifty-four minutes. What a great feeling.

It was a special accomplishment, but I hesitated to celebrate too much or too soon since I didn't know where Sabrina was on the course. One by the one, the minutes ticked by. And after ten minutes passed and she hadn't come in yet, I started to get a little concerned. A few more minutes passed until I was put at ease. I saw her round the corner and approach the finish line. She looked to be in pain from last weekend's fall, but she was still running and still smiling. Done!

Sabrina was a little disappointed that she didn't achieve the time she was hoping for. But in my mind, I thought it was exceptional that she even showed up to the start line, nevertheless had finished the race in a respectable time. On top of being my hero for getting back on her horse a week earlier, Sabrina was my rockstar wife, who completed her first half-marathon in just over two hours.

Sabrina and I have always been more than just a married couple. We're blessed to be the best and proudest of friends. The only thing greater than seeing your best friend and love accomplish feats of greatness like this is seeing your children do it. Life presented Sabrina with an additional challenge to overcome, and she rose to accomplish her goal with a smile. What another great example for our girls.

As we turned the calendar over to October, everything in our lives seemed to be going according to plan. Sabrina and I were in the best shape of our lives and enjoyed spending much of our time outdoors. That summer, I had also purchased a new carbon road bicycle and had enjoyed getting out for the occasional two- or three-hour rides with my buddies. Getting stronger and faster felt wonderful. Having completed the Oakville Half-Marathon on Labour Day weekend, I was riding a high. All cylinders were firing, and I had this confidence that I could accomplish anything I set my mind to.

Looking at the list from New Year's Eve, Sabrina and I had accomplished nearly all of our goals. I knew we still had a few more months to finish out the year, but rather than worrying about the odd item that I hadn't achieved yet in 2008, I was already thinking about the list we were going to create for 2009. All the incredible things we could do, especially with the girls growing older and being so adventurous.

As I suspect most dads do, I wanted to share all my passions with Chloe and Zara. Riding bikes, camping, playing soccer, building forts, going for nature hikes and building things in my workshop were top of my list. I'd already introduced these activities and sports to the girls, but it was always in short snippets, understanding that they were still very young. I was determined to help the girls with whatever interested them, and with a little luck, we'd have lots of things in common that we enjoy doing together for life. What more could I ask for? I had three beautiful girls, a career that was taking off, a lovely home and a fantastic family and group of friends. Life was good, and I knew it.

Maybe it was too good.

Chapter 2
One Day in the Woods

There are few things in life that I enjoy more than motorcycling. One of my earliest memories is going for a ride on my uncle Tom's Triumph. I was only a child and sat on the tank with my hands on the bars in front of me. The colours, the chrome, the smell, the sounds, the power—it only took 100 metres of going up and down my street once. I was hooked for life.

When I was seventeen, I finally had enough money to purchase my first motorcycle, but having older brothers and cousins with minibikes allowed me to occasionally twist a throttle in my backyard to keep the dream of motorcycling alive. For the day-to-day of normal life, though, I truly felt that the next best thing to a motorcycle was a bicycle. From my earliest memory of riding whatever bike my brothers left lying around the house (some without brakes), I lived on two wheels exploring all around my neighbourhood and the park across from our home. A bicycle was freedom and independence, and as long as I was home for dinner, I could venture as far as my legs would take me.

From the age of 17 to my early 30s, any time that I spent on two wheels involved motors. Road, dirt, the racetrack; it was the best. Around the age of 35, living in Oakville and close to some nice forest trails, I decided to get back into cycling. Mountain bikes had come a long way since I was young, so I found a nice quality hardtail with front suspension. Getting out into the forest with friends brought back fond memories and a way to make new ones. Like most people, I think I've always enjoyed the feeling of getting stronger and faster with each ride, as well as the camaraderie of riding in a close formation or drafting one another. And, of course, conquering a hill or obstacle in the forest that looks nearly impossible.

October 5th, 2008, was a Sunday. Around 7:00 AM, I ventured to the trail behind my house and waited for my friend, Eric, and a few of his neighbours to ride by so I could join them. It was a perfect day. We planned to hit the trails early so we could be back at home in time to have breakfast with our families by 9:00. Eric and the boys showed up, and we set out for the Bronte Creek trail.

Eric also worked at Microsoft, and through mountain biking, we developed a friendship. It was Eric and his neighbours that started the Sunday morning rides about a year before, and he generously let me join them.

The sun rose slowly, warming the cool air and evaporating the dew on everything. We were going to get wet and muddy from the look of the sky, but that would just make the ride more memorable. Plus, I'd be able to chase my girls around the house with the threat of a muddy hug when I got home. Chloe and Zara just loved it when I did that. They'd see me at the back door threatening to come in all dirty, and when I threw open the door and ran inside, they took off as fast as their little feet could go. Giggling and squealing and laughing, this was as much fun for me as the entire bike ride.

Chloe, the older sister, had always been sweet and kind, with a quiet confidence and steely determination. As her dad, I marvelled at her ability to keenly observe any person or situation before making a move and then moving with precision and fortitude. If something interested Chloe, she'd not stop until she achieved perfection. If there was a group of children, she would find a way to be its leader. And should there be a moment when she wasn't busy perfecting something, you'd find her coming in for a cuddle. She was such a great kid and an amazing big sister to Zara.

Born 26 months after Chloe, I'd best describe Zara as our firecracker. Zara didn't just look up to Chloe; she looked beyond her. Whatever Chloe did, Zara was determined to try and do it as well or better. Academics, riding a bike, soccer, playing piano, riding ponies… Zara was a force to be reckoned with. Consequently, it was only natural that when I came home all muddy from my ride and the great chase was about to begin, Zara was right beside her big sister, ready to fully participate in the fun.

Because it was later in the season, we were all in good shape for mountain biking. So, the pace was fast, and we made quick work of the roads leading to the main trail along the Creek. In no time at all, we stopped at one of the major roads that intersect the trail. We caught our breath and decided which way to go next. Two of the guys were tight for time that day, so they headed back home and left us to venture on. Eric and I discussed the options of where to ride. We could go either across the road into the tight, twisty trail or take a right and make our way to a creek a few kilometres to the east. Because I had done the route to the creek a few days before with my cousin, I suggested we try something different and cross into the forest. The trails I wanted were quite technical. I likened them to a playground of paths and obstacles that snake back and forth throughout the forest. Eric was always up for some fun, so away we went.

Earlier in the season, these technical trails were a bigger challenge. Of course, it didn't help that I had been a bit out of shape from eating all winter. One Sunday during the summer, I remember both Eric and me trying to complete an obstacle at the bottom of the hill that involved cycling up a 2x6-inch board onto a large, fallen tree. We had been three feet off the ground and riding along slippery wood, attempting to reach the ramp at the far side. Eric tried it and fell off the first time. I tried and got halfway along before I got scared of slipping and bunny-hopped off. Eric went again and made it all the way. I tried again and went for it. *Wham!* My front wheel slipped off, and I landed chest-first on the log. I collected myself quickly and decided to call it a day. Nothing injured but my pride. I told myself I'd try again sometime when the top of the log wasn't as slippery.

It was a kilometre or two through thick bush to get to our intended area. The technical trails and obstacles were beautiful. After five or ten minutes, we cycled through a small stream and then hugged the side of a hill under a canopy of low-hanging branches. Rounding the hill through this tunnel of dense foliage, the path opened to a clearing where I saw something unexpected. On the long, steep downhill in front of us, a tree had fallen across the path. And on this downed tree, someone had built a ramp.

If you ride a bike, you've fallen off a bike. That's the trade-off involving anything with two wheels, and it's a risk I was generally okay with. We went to the forest to play. And when I came across this new ramp on the hill, I wanted to give it a try. With a bit of luck, it would be another thing for me to know that I could do.

Whoever built the ramp made it run level from five feet before the fallen tree and then a couple of feet beyond, creating a four-foot drop at the end of the platform.

Eric mentioned that he and the guys saw the ramp last weekend, but none of them had dared to try it. Trying to be brave, I acknowledged what I thought was the worst-case scenario and said, "You might need to help me get out of here if I break my bike."

I never thought for a second that I might hurt myself, and it's not because I've never been hurt. As an adult playing sports and riding motorcycles, I've broken a few bones. Wrist, hand, shoulder, and of course, my collarbone. It was a consequence of "going for it," and I'd always been comfortable that the risks were worth the experience. If I contemplated the potential of injuring myself, it was never anything more serious than a broken limb. Time and hard work—and maybe physiotherapy in the worst case—would get my health back should an accident happen. Having raced (and crashed) motorcycles at over 150 km/h, there was not a lot that scared me, and I certainly wasn't concerned about this simple jump in the forest.

I rode up the hill a short distance and turned around to hit the ramp. As I coasted along the platform, I started to gain an appreciation for the height at the end. I was a little surprised how high it felt but kept going anyway. As I came to the end, I was moving slowly and knew that I didn't have enough speed to land partway down the hill, so I decided at the last second to bunny-hop off of it. This had worked in the past and should be fine.

But things were different this time. Unlike when I'd hopped off the other obstacles, this time, my bike starts to tip forward in the air so that instead of landing on both wheels at the same time, I land on the front wheel. Looking back, I should have thrown away the bike and protected myself. But instead, I hold on to the handlebars and wait for my back tire to hit the ground so I can carry on down the hill.

The back tire doesn't fall. Instead, I tip forward over the front of the handlebars, and my head plows into the ground. I hear my back snap as my legs fall over my head. FUCK!

I tried to sit up but couldn't. I tried to move my legs but couldn't. I reached down to check that my lower half was still there. It was, but while my brain was sending the right signals, nothing happened.

I yelled to Eric, "I can't feel my legs!"

He ran over in a panic and asked if I had my cell phone. I didn't, and neither did he. So, he jumped on his bike and raced back to the road to get help.

I was all by myself, lying on this hill, staring up into the canopy as the morning sun tried desperately to shine through. Everything was completely still, including me.

As I laid there, my mind started to race and ask itself questions in some primal sort of rapid-fire-crisis-problem-solving way. *If I've broken my back, how will I be able to dance with my little girls when they get married? How will I live in my two-story home? It has stairs. How will I ride my motorcycle? How will I play with the girls? How will I continue my career with Microsoft?*

But the question that hits me the hardest is, *What have I just done to Sabrina? She married an active guy. How is this going to impact her?* I was scared.

My mind scurried in every direction. I knew this was bad. I knew I must figure out how to minimize the negative impact of this on me, my family, and my friends. I wasn't crying yet; I had to be in a state of shock and, honestly, I had too much shit to figure out. I needed answers for the endless list of questions that poured into my head. FUCK!

The answers weren't coming to me. I wanted my head to clear so I could think, but it was overloaded, trying to process too much too quickly.

Oh, shit, I thought. *I'm supposed to be in Toronto later today for my IT security conference. I can't let my friends down.* For a second, I thought that maybe with a little luck, I'd just miss that night, and I could make up for it on Monday and Tuesday. I didn't want to inconvenience anyone.

The emergency personnel were taking time. *Where are they? Where is Eric?* I started shivering uncontrollably. The cold of the forest floor combined with my body going into shock began to take over.

Back to problem-solving, but my mind was all over the place. Trying to strategize solutions to every little problem I could think of was impossible. I had no idea of the depth and complexity of challenges that I was going to be faced with. Then it occurred to me: *Maybe I should try to think of new opportunities that this might create. If I'm off work for a period of time, maybe I could take more piano lessons.* Immediately following this thought, I realized that I needed my feet for the pedals, so that wouldn't work. I remembered watching the Paralympics during the summer. Maybe there was a sport I could do to get me there. That'd be cool.

As for my career, I told myself that this didn't have to be the end. I could keep my goals. I just needed to acknowledge that they'd be harder to achieve and would likely take longer too. I entertained the idea that completing anything without the use of my legs should be more rewarding and satisfying, but only time would tell.

The pain came on in waves. I was so cold. I just wanted to be warm and home and with my girls. I listened for Eric, for help, for anybody, but the forest was dead quiet. I couldn't help but think that the forest was so beautiful, and I was so damaged... Helpless. What had I done?

The first to arrive were the paramedics, and they were breathing heavily. I suppose that it was to be expected as they just hiked deep into the forest with all their equipment. As the one guy sorted out his gear, he started peppering me with questions. What's your name, where are you, what happened, can I cut off your clothes and test you for feeling?

I assumed he started at my feet and worked his way up my body. "Can you feel this? Can you feel this? How about now?" When he got to my chest, midway between my belly button and chest, I felt something. He drew a line on my skin with a marker so they could see at the hospital if the paralysis was getting better or worse with time. This was not good.

One by one, Eric brought the rescue personnel to me. It was getting busy with what looked like paramedics, firemen, police, and even a reporter taking pictures. All of them were asking me questions and trying to size up the situation. I heard a couple of them discussing the easiest way to get me out of the forest. If they could get me up the steep hill, they could walk through the farmer's field and bring me to the helicopter that was on its way to take me to Hamilton General Hospital.

After what seemed like thirty minutes, they had their plan. A group of them counted down from three and then lifted me onto a flat board. The pain was indescribable. Whereas the contour of the ground seemed to somewhat accommodate having two of my vertebrae on top of each other, the flat stretcher accentuated the injury and the intensity of the pain. It got even worse when they strapped me down so tight that I was essentially one with the board. After some more discussion, six of them lifted me off the ground and started plodding up the hill. There were three on each side of me; I couldn't help but liken this to pallbearers carrying a casket.

They decided not to follow the bike path that they took to reach me. Rather, we headed straight up the hill, through the thickest part of the forest where no path existed. For some reason, someone thought this was a better option, but I wasn't so sure. I think they thought that if we could just get out of the forest and into the farmer's field at the top of the hill, the helicopter could pick me up from there.

These were details I could care less about. I was consumed by the pain searing through my body with every step they took. I thought I had a good tolerance for pain, but this was beyond anything I'd ever experienced before in my life.

In an attempt to ease the pain, even just for a second, I tried moaning. Then I tried breathing out. I started crying… nothing helped.

Any previous illusions I might have had that this might not be too serious were dashed with a look at my rescuers' faces. They averted their eyes, but the gravity of my situation was visible on their faces. Navigating a path through the forest up a steep hill was a challenge at the best of times. To do it while carrying an adult man on a stretcher was another thing entirely.

At the top of the hill, I heard them say that they still had to carry me all the way to the parking lot because the helicopter pilot wasn't comfortable landing in the field. He didn't like the look of the ground covered with cut-down corn stocks and would prefer to land on the hard-packed parking lot. Of course, I didn't realize it in the moment, but my life moving forward would forever be preoccupied with having to be concerned about the ground surface I needed to wheel on.

It was around that time that one of the men carrying me started to complain about the difficulty of walking through the field, carrying me. *Are you fucking kidding me?* I thought to myself. *You're carrying a guy who will likely never walk again, and you're complaining about how hard it is to carry me, with five other men? What an ass.*

Eventually, we made it to the helicopter, and I was transferred in. The paramedics were all business and tended to their jobs of monitoring my status while the pilot flew us to the hospital. My head must have still been taped to the flat board. All I can remember seeing is the ceiling of the helicopter as the deafening noise of the engines and rotors roared.

I asked for something for the pain but was denied. The intensity and volume of pain I experienced seemed to force me in and out of consciousness. Upon landing, we were quickly brought into some kind of ER waiting room. The nurses wanted to remove my wedding ring, but they were unable to get it over my knuckle. They suggested cutting it off, but I wouldn't let them. It was too special, and it was too symbolic; there was no way I was going to let anyone destroy it. "Find some lube!" I instructed them.

I was still shaking and so very cold. I asked for blankets, but instead, the nurses put a plastic blanket over me and started pumping hot air under it to try and warm me. Only years later did I learn that they should have been doing the exact opposite, putting me in a tub of ice water to slow down the swelling where my back was broken and pumping me full of cold IV. Yes, they were trying to warm me like I asked. But this likely made my spinal cord injury worse, as the swelling moved up my spine, killing all of the nerves one vertebra at a time.

Before long, Sabrina arrived. She looked confused as I shivered under the blanket, crying. All I could do was apologize to her over and over again. "I'm so sorry, I'm so sorry," I just keep repeating. She had no idea what happened. The police had come to the house and told her that I was in an accident, and she needed to come to the hospital, but they didn't provide any details. They offered to drive her, but she preferred to drive herself. She assumed I had broken my wrist or my shoulder or something else less catastrophic.

As time passed, some of my friends showed up at the hospital as well. Eric and his wife, Lucy, came and comforted me while I waited to be brought into surgery. I kept falling in and out of consciousness, and at some point, I must have been sedated for my operation. Because when I awoke, I found myself in what looked like the ICU. But I wasn't really sure where I was.

Chapter 3

Doctors and Hospitals

I awoke from surgery to find a doctor at the foot of my bed, looking at an x-ray of what I assumed was my spine. I could see vertebrae on top of each other on the screen. It didn't look good, but still, I asked him how bad it was. He responded, "You're lucky to be alive."

That hit me hard. Everything before this moment felt like chaos, but those words left no ambiguity as to my situation. If I wasn't going to be able to walk, I needed to get back to the problem-solving I was doing in the forest. I had to salvage my future. I suppose, in theory, there was a decision to be made with regards to how I was going to respond to this new reality, but for me, it was a no-brainer; I was going to make the best of whatever ability I still had. That's just the way I'm hardwired. Being jaded and miserable wouldn't help anyone, especially me and my girls, so I decided to focus on being grateful I was alive and could still move my upper body. It could have been so much worse. If I were going to get through this, it would be on focusing on how lucky I was, even if I couldn't walk.

Those first few days in the ICU were a blur. I spent more time asleep than awake, and when I was conscious, it was likely because I was being taken for an x-ray or scan. Being moved around and forced to sit up for the x-rays was excruciating. I'd often wake to find a different family member or friend at my bedside and did my best to acknowledge and interact with whoever had been kind enough to visit me. All the while struggling to comprehend the extent of what had happened.

A day or two after my surgery, I woke to find my manager from work and my mother-in-law beside my bed. These weren't two people I expected to see here together, though I was appreciative. My mother-in-law didn't say much. She looked pissed, and honestly, I couldn't really blame her. I knew she wanted what was best for her daughter and grandchildren, and me hurting myself in a catastrophic way put our future in question. The idea of having a paraplegic son-in-law must have been almost as unknown and scary to her as it was to me.

My manager didn't make the situation better when he asked me, "Rob, tell me, is it true that you took a ten-foot jump?" I didn't even need to look at my mother-in-law to feel her glare intensify at the thought. Sunday had been both her wedding anniversary and her husband's birthday. Obviously, I messed up her special day in an epic way, not to mention potentially messing up her daughter's life.

"No, no," I explained to him. "It was more like three or four feet." As if that might somehow sound better and more responsible to my mother-in-law. I wanted her to know that I hadn't been blatantly careless. This jump should have been doable, and it certainly was not something that I considered to be potentially life-changing. I took the chance to look her in the eyes, but once more, I got nothing from her but a cold stare. Again, I couldn't really blame her.

My life was a series of little moments like this. In the ICU, my world was a jambalaya of sleep, pain, short visits and tests. Family, friends, and doctors—all of them had my best interests at heart.

While I tried to be composed and keep my shit together on the outside, inside, I was struggling to make some sense of my new reality.

As the days slowly passed, I lost track of how many times a day I was taken to the pit of the hospital for an x-ray or CT scan. If I didn't have to sit up in bed so they could see my chest properly, I probably wouldn't have cared. But it was so painful each time. Unbearable pain. After a few days of this, I spoke up and asked why so many tests needed to be performed. It was then a nurse told me that the doctors were concerned that I might have also broken my neck and that they were monitoring the blood building up around my lungs. As it turned out, when I fell, I also punctured my lung.

When the day came to move out of the ICU, I thought it must have been a good thing but knew that only time would tell. Flanked by Sabrina and my brother-in-law, Amir, a person from the hospital moved my bed to the Spinal Cord Injury (SCI) recovery wing. It took place during a shift change, so while there was a lot of movement going on all around me, I wasn't engaged by any of the nurses. In fact, I kind of felt like I was purposely being ignored. For a moment, I wondered if I should tell them to take me back to the ICU. There I received a lot of support and attention.

In my new room, after what felt like a couple of hours, a nurse finally came around to check on me. I asked everyone who interacted with me for their name and if they knew the particulars about my injury and prescribed care, but it was useless. Not only were these nurses unaware of my pain protocol—established and refined in the ICU—but they seemed ambivalent to what I was going through. Frustrated and exhausted, I hoped I could just sleep the rest of the day away and that tomorrow would be better.

Sleep came after receiving my pain meds. But I was startled awake during the night when an alarm on the machine that dispenses my pain meds started blaring. It turned out no one plugged this machine in when I was moved, and the battery was almost dead. Looking for the call button to notify the nurses, I discovered I wasn't given one of those either. This was not good. I thought to myself, *Come on, people, get your shit together.*

This experience confirmed that I would have been better off left in the ICU. Here in this unit, the hospital staff were just overwhelmed and consumed with the needs and requests of the other three people in my room and those throughout the floor who were in worse shape or simply more demanding. Unless I had a pressing issue that required immediate attention and an alarm went off or I spoke out, I'd have to figure things out for myself or just suck it up.

On my second day outside of the ICU, I asked the nurses if I could speak to the surgeon who performed my operation. I wanted to learn how the surgery went and ask him some questions about my recovery. It took a few hours, which was fine, but when he arrived at my bedside, he stood there like a robot. Cold as stone. I began asking him questions and every answer he gave was one word accompanied by a blank stare. No explanations, no details, no comforting, no bedside manner. What a dick.

He seemed puzzled as to why I would ask all these questions and why I started becoming agitated with his demeanour. As my frustration grew, I started crying. I was so confused and sad. *What the fuck is wrong with this man?* I questioned. When he left my room, I shared my frustration with the nurses and supervisors. They seemed to bite their tongues, not wanting to say too much about a doctor, but they nodded in agreement with the specifics of my rant. And it was apparent that they felt unable to do anything to change him, even if they wanted to.

After a few hours, I was approached by someone from the hospital holding a clipboard with a document on it that she asked me to sign. I asked what it was for and was told that it would allow the hospital to conduct an HIV test. "Why?" I asked, more than a little confused. The person told me that during surgery, one of the students operating the power drill used to install the hardware in my back slipped with the drill and cut themselves.

Are you fucking kidding me? Is it training week in the hospital, and students are learning how to use power tools on my spine? How the hell does this happen? And while we're on the subject of HIV, how do I know that I'm not the one that's been compromised by the student? It's not like me to get angry, but I felt it coming on. In my head, I thought, *Get me out of this fucking room. Get me out of this fucking hospital.* If I had more energy and fewer filters, I'd have started ripping people new ones. It's probably for the best that I didn't. Instead, I signed the permission form and went back to focusing on trying to escape from the intense pain of being alive and breathing.

A day later, I transferred to a semi-private room. "A room with a view" is what my friends called it, as there was a window beside my bed overlooking part of Hamilton. The city isn't that attractive, but the sunshine was encouraging. This was a much better room to have visitors in, too. Which was good because when the permission was given to have visitors, they started coming in droves. That made me happy.

My brother-in-law Amir flew up from his home in Los Angeles when he heard the news and stayed with me day and night. Amir is

Sabrina's younger brother. We met when Sabrina and I started dating, and right from the beginning, I knew that he would be an important part of my life. Someone I should definitely watch and learn from. Amir's unique blend of charm and intellect distinguished him from anyone else I knew. And while I hoped that over the years I might contribute to his life, I was quite sure I'd come out ahead for having him in mine. I loved him like a brother. And, true to form, it was no surprise that when I had my accident, he immediately jumped on a plane to come and help us out.

Having Amir in the hospital with me was comforting and helpful, but after a few days, I had to insist that he take a break and go home with Sabrina to have a proper night's sleep. A week or so into my hospital stay, two friends from work came by and brought me a very thoughtful gift. In addition to a framed picture of the two of them posing, which just made me laugh (and hurt from the movement of laughing), they pulled out of their gift bag a thin white sheet of plastic that stuck to the wall with static and dry erase markers. They told me that when Chloe and Zara came to visit, they'd be able to draw on the plastic. What a thoughtful gift.

Later that day, my primary doctor came to check on me. Amir was back, and he put the plastic on the wall and started writing down what the doctor told me about my injury, prognosis, and treatment/pain protocol. I now had my chart on the wall in front of my bed that included when I could expect the next round of meds and painkillers, as well as other important information. Within a day, the plastic was filled with notes, so Sabrina brought in large sheets of paper that she and Amir could tape to the wall. This was a powerful thing for me. I had access to my chart, and I could ensure the hospital staff gave me the proper care that was most recently prescribed.

Having something written to reference, I could call out any of the mistakes or inconsistencies the staff were making.

Not surprisingly, the doctors and nurses appeared to have mixed feelings about my wall chart. I had taken back a small amount of control over my care and wasn't shy to question things, regardless of whom I was speaking to. One example of the power of this info happened when the night nurse handed me a little dispensing cup with my medications in it. When I compared what was in the cup to the list of prescribed meds that was on my wall chart, I noticed that my painkillers were missing. With every breath I took, it hurt. I needed my pain meds. I asked her why the painkillers were missing, and she told me that it was because she was going from memory based on yesterday's meds. She admitted that someone else had my chart, and rather than look for it, she just relied on her memory.

It isn't the case that the people working in the hospital are lazy or incompetent. Far from it, but they have to deliver incredibly complex care under serious time and resource constraints. By then, I knew too well that mistakes happen, and I tried to be patient while also advocating for myself. But if I ever had a doubt before entering the hospital that it was crucial to own your own care, that doubt was now gone.

The days started to tick by. When I was alone, most of my waking moments were filled with this odd combination of fear, sadness, and impatience. I felt like a prisoner in the bed, and I desperately wanted to get out of the hospital to start my recovery. I wanted to prove to myself, my girls, and the world that I was okay.

Nurses and doctors checked on me throughout the day and night, but they never lingered. There was only enough time for one or two questions before they carried on with their rounds. The hospital was a factory of illness and injury, and I was just one of many needing their attention. I learned to be the squeaky wheel when I really needed something, but my preference would have been to not be there at all. I was the person who loved to help others, so having to ask for help—even if it was medical staff in a hospital—wasn't something that I was good at. I think I knew this was going to have to change, but it sucked on so many levels, and I was going to fight it.

In addition to the stream of doctors and nurses that checked on me, there was a woman assigned to help me navigate the additional challenges of learning to live with a spinal cord injury. Before my accident, I didn't know anyone who was paraplegic. I knew you couldn't walk but never really thought about the other challenges paraplegics must deal with. I was forced to learn quickly.

I appreciated this woman being available to help Sabrina and me, but the way she spoke down to me was difficult to handle. It was hard to pinpoint one thing about her. But for starters, the way she slowed down her speaking and tried to oversimplify everything was just brutal. I asked her repeatedly to speed up and get to the heart of the matter that she was trying to convey, as I struggled to stay awake as she spoke. I avoided saying out loud the thoughts going on in my head, which was *I have a four- and two-year-old at home, so please stop talking to me like I'm a child.* I wanted her to jump to the important parts quickly. Specifically, how do I fix this? *Shit, lady! I've broken my back, not my head, and I don't need anyone talking down to me.* I didn't appreciate the condescension.

I told myself that she meant well, yet I couldn't get over feeling insulted. Is this what I should expect now that I'm in a wheelchair? And if a professional who specializes in working with people with spinal cord injuries is speaking like this to me, what can I expect from the general public? I desperately wanted to tell her: "Know your audience and speak to them accordingly. Otherwise, you're going to piss a lot of people off." Not unlike how she had me feeling in that moment.

It was around this time in the hospital that I learned more about the technical specifics of the spinal cord. The vertebrae in your spine are grouped into sections, and the higher the level of injury, the more ability you are likely to lose. Starting at the neck, you have the cervical nerves, which are numbered C1 through C8. If you break C1 or C2, right at the very top, you're probably dead. Below the cervical nerves are the thoracic nerves, which is where my break occurred. I broke T11/T12, which is near the bottom of this section. A lot of people in my situation would still be able to feel and control their bowel or bladder and might even have sexual function. For me, though, the additional damage to my spinal cord that happened with the swelling after my accident, and any of the damage caused by the slipping of the drill during the operation, resulted in my final paralysis going up to T7. So, whenever someone hears that I broke T11/T12, there is always an assumption that I have more physical ability than I actually do.

For all my frustrations within the hospital, I did consider myself fortunate that there were some quality caregivers to help me. One nurse in the ICU stood above the rest. Her name escapes me, but I remember her sweet voice and how she took a few minutes each shift to hold my hand and assure me that I was going to be okay and accomplish great things. Her kindness and thoughtfulness touched me. She was a bright light in a dark sea of overworked caregivers.

In addition to breaking my back, my punctured lung was a growing concern. While the stream of visitors was wonderful, I found my health deteriorating and breathing more difficult each day. Out of the blue, I was struck with the fear that because I was weak and having trouble breathing, that I might be developing pneumonia. Flashing back to my father-in-law, who was fighting lung cancer when pneumonia took his life, I couldn't help but worry that something like that could happen to me in my weakened state. I knew I was expending a lot of energy with my visitors, so we decided to ask everyone to stay away for a few days so I could focus on resting and healing.

The combination of my increasing pain and difficulty breathing resulted in the recommendation to insert a chest tube. This tube would allow the fluid pushing on my lungs to drain so that my lungs could heal and fully expand again.

The doctor explained the procedure, assuring me that it was simple, short, and implying that it wouldn't be too painful. I agreed immediately as it sounded like a proven solution to make my breathing easier and to accelerate my recovery. Usually, I'm suspicious of anything that sounds too easy or good to be true. My decision to move forward with doing this was undoubtedly influenced by the doctor being young, charismatic, and brimming with confidence.

Unfortunately, the reality of the procedure was considerably different from what I was told (or, one might say, "sold"). The first thing the doctor did was numb the area where the tube enters my body, injecting the syringe just under the surface where the incision will be made. I looked away and focused on my breathing, knowing that on a breath out, the pain seemed to disappear or at least lessen significantly. Slow, deep breaths, in and out. Next, the doctor made the movement of putting down the syringe and picking up what I assumed was a scalpel. I was still looking away, but as he was right over me, I couldn't help but see him from the corner of my eye.

If the needle to numb the skin was an eight out of ten on the pain scale, as I continued to look to the left of my bed, the pain I started feeling was suddenly an eleven! The breathing trick no longer helped. My brain wouldn't fall for it anymore; it was on high alert and wanted me to find the source of this pain so I could stop it. More pain. More pain. More pain. I couldn't look away any longer, so I turned to where the pain emanated. What I saw was chilling.

Looking down at the right side of my chest, I saw the doctor's gloved hand pull back slowly, revealing a blood-covered finger from inside my chest. What the fuck?! In addition to the bloodied glove, the slurping sound of his finger exiting the incision made me shiver.

"I need to be careful not to allow more air in," he said as he reached for the chest tube from his surgical tray and started feeding it back into the hole he had just made. Through skin, muscle and other tissue that he just tore open using his finger! Fuck me! No wonder it hurt like a son-of-a-bitch. I wanted to punch the bastard.

I told him how much it hurt, and the fucker said quite simply and almost cheerfully, "Don't worry, I've done this procedure before many times." That does not help me. I asked him if he's ever done this in a way that wasn't so painful to the patient or if he had ever experienced the procedure himself? He replied with a smart-ass remark. I was so pissed. What the fuck!?

Inch by inch, I saw and felt him pushing the tube into my body. He seemed pleased with himself, as if he finally got to do an exciting procedure for a change. He was indifferent to my experience but seemed happy as though everything (from his perspective) was going to plan. I looked away again, this time in disgust and frustration. It was probably best not to watch, as he told me he just stitched the tube to my skin and taped everything down with layers of tape across my chest, sides, and into my armpits to keep it all in place. With every breath I took, my lungs expanded and pushed against the tube. This just made the pain worse.

A day passed, and I tried hard to be brave and suck up the pain, but it was the worst it had been since the forest. I asked every doctor that checked on me to make it better, but all they seemed interested in doing was playing with the dosage or type of painkiller. Some meds made me itchy; others made me nauseated. The doctors pretended to be making progress at finding the exact right cocktail that would help me, but with each shift change, it felt more and more like they were just freestyling with my meds until they got to go home. I was stuck there, and I was hurting.

Day two of the chest tube was even worse. In this odd state of what seemed like being in and out of consciousness, I couldn't stay awake because I was so exhausted from the pain, but I couldn't sleep soundly either because the pain kept me awake. My siblings, mom, and other close friends and family checked on me and spent their entire visit just massaging my neck and scratching my head. Anything to provide me with a little relief, but the pain persisted. And I was mostly silent.

I felt bad for not being a good host to those who'd taken time to visit with me. Fortunately, I knew they understood, and they seemed happy to be able to comfort me, even if it was just a little. I was so grateful to have so many friends and family showing me their kindness.

On Friday, the day before Thanksgiving, the nurses and doctors had a detectable spring in their step. They all seemed excited about the upcoming long weekend and appeared to be in a rush to get through rounds, meaning they spent even less time with each of their patients.

Made aware of the state I was in, the young doctor who had inserted the chest tube—you'll remember him as "the fucker"—came to see me. Conceding that perhaps he pushed the tube in a little too far, he suggested trying to pull it back an inch or two to see if that would lessen the pain when I breathed. I gave him permission to try.

Unfortunately, moving the chest tube meant peeling off the multiple layers of tape from my chest and cutting the stitches that were holding the tube in place. The stitches weren't a big deal, but peeling off the tape was excruciatingly painful. Why on Earth did he run tape into my armpit hair? I couldn't think of any reason why a sane person would do this to another, let alone a "caregiver" doing it. This just further cemented my opinion that this doctor was a fucking prick.

After the tape and stitches were removed, he tugged on the tube, pulling it back an inch or two, and then proceeded to tape everything all over again. It felt like the end of the tube was in a different spot, but the pain wasn't any less.

The next day the pain hadn't subsided one bit. I was beside myself, and Sabrina and Amir could see it. They escalated my concerns yet again until we finally got some action.

Dr. Karen, the on-call anesthesiologist, introduced herself. She'd learned that I was in terrible pain and wanted to help. "There's no reason for you to be in such agony," she said. In short order, Dr.

Karen performed a nerve block between my ribs that numbed my torso and allowed the pain I was experiencing to decrease from an eleven out of ten to about a three. I was happy with three. I could now eat, sleep, and just be without the blinding waves of pain that previously shocked me with every breath. The next day, as the nerve block started to wear off, a second on-call anesthesiologist performed the procedure again to allow me to get through the weekend.

On Monday, my nurse held up the bag that had been collecting blood and fluid from my lungs. The draining appeared to have stopped. The bag was very full. She told me the doctors expected to capture half a litre of blood and fluid, but it turned out we collected nearly two litres. While there was some comfort to know that all this had truly been necessary, these last few days had been the most painful of my life.

I hoped things would improve moving forward. With the pain manageable again and my lungs cleared, I could now focus less on surviving and more on my rehabilitation—and, of course, my guests.

Chapter 4

This Guy Can Fly

After having the chest tube finally removed and being able to breathe more comfortably once again, things started to improve a little. Family and friends filled my room and made moments better. Some of my visitors liked to just hold my hand. Others stood away from my bed, feeling terrible for me that I broke my back and digging deep to hold back their tears. Fortunately, most were full of smiles and laughter as they successfully lifted my spirits while at the same time trying to assess how Sabrina and I were dealing with our new reality.

My roommate was an older gentleman who seemed fine with all of the traffic and noise coming from my side of the room; he even joined in some of the conversations. He was there for foot and ankle surgery after breaking both when the extension ladder he was standing on slipped and fell to the ground. Even though Chloe and Zara were a little tentative coming to visit me in the hospital, they were kind to my roommate. And he clearly enjoyed their presence in our room. My favourite part was when they climbed onto my bed and gave me cuddles. For those precious minutes, I could close my eyes, and life felt normal, and I felt whole again. I didn't want them to ever leave.

A friend brought in a high-speed wireless access router and set it up in the window, allowing me to get online for the first time since the accident. In 2008 you were not allowed to have your cell phones turned on within the hospital, so having a way to get online and connect with the world was great.

Amir started a blog that Sabrina would update daily, sharing what was happening at home and the hospital. It was an efficient way to update a lot of people quickly and at our convenience. As a bonus, it was also a good place for those thinking of visiting to see when a good time might be, without having to speak directly to Sabrina. Just a few days after launching the website, the daily volume of traffic was in the tens of thousands. Either I knew a lot of people who cared about me, or bad news and drama was fodder for the masses. I think it was a little of both.

I've always found it an odd thing that when tragedy strikes an individual or family, the ones trying to catch their breath and recover are also the ones most expected to comfort everyone around them. My accident was no different. I was grateful for the countless number of people genuinely concerned about my family and me and understood that they wanted to know details about what was happening and how I was going to be. Many also wanted to know how they could help. The blog was a good way for people to get that info and provide comfort without putting Sabrina through the emotional stress of telling everyone the same thing countless times a day. She was busy with two young girls, preparing our home for a renovation to make it accessible, and visiting me in the hospital. Updates needed to be efficient, and I think people realized that we were getting on with things as best we could.

In addition to keeping everyone informed, the blog also provided me with a lot of inspiration and encouragement to recover. Being able to read the good wishes, and responding to them when I had the energy, focus, and desire to do so, was invaluable. Technology had always been a big part of my life leading up to the accident, so it was no surprise that from day one of my recovery, it had continued to be.

I wasn't able to leave my bed, but technology let me stay connected to the world. A world that, by virtue of my injury, was now very different than the one I was used to.

The moments when my pain was manageable, and I was all alone, my thoughts and internet searches focused on trying to educate and prepare myself for life as a paraplegic. Beyond no longer being able to walk, I was trying to anticipate all the new firsts in the coming days and months that I wanted to accomplish. Being a good dad, living in my home, going for my first drive, my first handcycle ride, how I might be able to swim, and on and on.

I was fortunate that the hospital had a professional peer support worker from Spinal Cord Injury Ontario who was able to share his experiences and knowledge of being paraplegic. I also leveraged Google to learn as much as I could. I'd type in search terms and add "+paraplegic" to see how others before me had done things. I needed information and examples to better understand and prepare for this new world, and the Internet didn't disappoint. There was so much material about diagnoses, treatments, and experiments to help me understand what to expect. I also found videos on YouTube of people with spinal cord injuries doing crazy shit and living large. This gave me hope for adventures still to come.

I was a newcomer to this world of paraplegia but was optimistic it could still be a world full of possibility and potential. Being able to speak with people who were already part of this world and having online access to learn and explore before I'd even left the hospital was indispensable. This allowed me to begin to understand that being paraplegic wasn't incompatible with having a good life and achieving my dreams. It was just going to be harder.

By the time I left Hamilton General, I was starting to have a better appreciation for the complexities that came with paraplegia. There were so many things that I never thought about, but of course, I never had a reason to. Beyond losing the ability to walk, I had to learn how to transfer from bed to chair and from chair to things like the shower bench or toilet. I learned how to dress myself, how to empty my bladder using a catheter (the short form is "IC," or intermittent catheterization), and how to empty my bowels. The most basic human functions that most of us take for granted, most of our lives, I had to learn all over again. With these new skills and finally stable enough to be transferred, I wanted to get the hell out of the hospital and take things to the next level. It was time for me to go to rehab.

Because my home is located between Toronto and Hamilton, I had the option of choosing which rehabilitation centre I wanted to go to. The facility in Hamilton is called Chedoke, and I was told that it was an older hospital that was soon to be replaced. The other option was Lyndhurst, near the Sunnybrook Hospital in Toronto. Friends took an afternoon to check out both facilities and came back saying there was simply no question where I should go—Lyndhurst.

I asked them for details on what they saw and learned at the two rehab centres. To my surprise, they had a lot to share. Having met with many support staff and being given tours of the facilities, they were visibly impressed with the resources available in Lyndhurst. They talked about feeling a positive energy to the place with people in wheelchairs zooming around in every direction. Upon being introduced to the staff, they were often asked what my level of injury was. When told T11, my friends were unanimously informed that I'd be jumping up and down curbs in my chair in no time at all. I took this to mean that I was lucky my injury wasn't higher and that in time I could be very capable and independent in my chair. It was late October now, and I was ready to make the trip to Lyndhurst to find out for myself.

The medical transport from Hamilton to Toronto was surprisingly painful. I felt every bump and crack in the road, and wow, there were so many. This experience made me grateful that I had been taken from the accident to the hospital in a helicopter.

Sabrina drove herself and beat us to Lyndhurst to start the checking-in process. With clinical efficiency, they took me up to my room on the second floor and transferred me from the ambulance stretcher to my new bed. I felt like a UPS package being moved around from building to vehicle to building with no say in the matter or very much interaction. I was repeatedly told to lay still, and everyone else would do all the work. It sucked.

I was genuinely excited to be leaving Hamilton General so that I could begin my rehab. I was eager to get to a facility that had the resources and people to teach me how to live without the use of my lower body. Unfortunately, I'd only been in my new bed for a few minutes when we started to smell an odour coming from my pants. After all the moving around, I had shit myself.

Damn it!

My first interactions with the nurses of Lyndhurst were them turning me over on my side and pulling shit out of my ass. I was embarrassed, helpless, and just so unbelievably sad. I'd had such high hopes going into rehab, so it was doubly devastating that my first experience had me in tears. The nurses probably didn't care, but I certainly did.

From the moment of my accident in the forest, I spent almost all my hours lying on my back and looking up. Four weeks in, and I'd begun to really hate the sight of ceiling tiles and fluorescent lights. They taunted me. I used to build suspended ceilings with my dad's construction business and took pride in calculating the dimensions and fitting together the puzzle of metal and tiles. Ceilings can be tedious work and always involve lots of ups and downs on the ladder. When I finished constructing a ceiling, I was happy it was done and in no rush to start another. But on this day, as I laid in another hospital bed staring at another ceiling, I became painfully aware that I'd never have the option again of building the things I used to.

Trying to settle into this new place, I kept my notebook handy and wrote down the things that I thought were important to the doctors and me. I noted body functions, how I was feeling, questions I had… those kinds of things. During the first few days, several different nurses and doctors came by my room to meet or check on me. I was trying to keep track of them all, but it was hard with the pace that they kept. They'd fly into my room, do something or ask me a question in a hurry, and then leave. No time for small talk or what I would call "caregiving." The way they treated me made me feel like a part on an assembly line. I tried to focus on the good, but it was hard.

After a couple of weeks at Lyndhurst, my frustration and anger towards the bulk of the nursing staff started to spike. Some mornings I'd wake up and, needing assistance from the nurses, I'd push the call button bell, only to see the light indicating that I had called them, cancelled. After ten minutes and no one coming, I'd push the button again, and again the light was turned off; no one came.

The first few times this happened, I told myself not to overreact and just let it go. No sense in pissing off my caregivers. But after the third or fourth time of this happening, I'd had it. Mad as hell, I used my pillow to snag my wheelchair and pull it beside my bed, did a controlled fall from the bed into my chair, and wheeled myself (in my underwear) to the nursing station. I sized up the situation and unleashed.

There were two nurses behind the desk, and neither of them would look at me as I spoke. I could even see that one was browsing the internet! After a couple of "Excuse me's" were ignored, I raised my voice, demanding to be acknowledged and looked at. I asked them why they continued to ignore the call button when I needed their help.

They said nothing, just stared blankly at me. No apology. Nothing. So, I spoke again… "Are you kidding me? If you're not going to help me when I need help, then why the hell am I here?"

Like the hospital, there were a few nurses at Lyndhurst who were really kind and experts at doing their jobs and being caregivers at the same time. But unfortunately, those good ones were the exception. At least half of the nursing staff that were assigned to me and my roommate ranged from cold and indifferent to outright cruel and abusive.

Some of the things I saw and heard from the nurses made me sad; other things just stirred my anger and frustration, like that one nurse in Lyndhurst who insisted that my roommate and I take lots of laxatives, regardless of our levels of injury. She threatened that if we didn't take as many laxatives as she told us to, that we risked vomiting our feces! While technically that is possible in the most extreme cases of constipation, the sad fact was that she just wanted my roommate to have softer stool so that her job would be easier when performing his bowel routine, and for me, she just simply didn't know or care that I was having the opposite problem. During my physiotherapy, when practicing transfers from the floor to my wheelchair, I often shit my pants. When I shared with my doctors what the nurse was saying, they just shook their heads and laughed it off. I think they had heard this before and found it funny.

The other extreme happened to me when a different nurse—who did learn that I was having bowel issues—insisted that I wasn't doing my own bowel routine properly and needed to be shown how to do it. She was adamant that she was going to show me how to do it properly, even though I couldn't understand how I would learn anything if I couldn't see or feel what was being done. I mean, seriously, I'm sticking my finger up my ass to pull the shit out. I think I can figure that out. Regardless, she said she could fix my problem, so I felt compelled to let her try. That evening, after doing her "thing," I transferred back to my wheelchair from the toilet to find the bowl full of my blood! In her haste to show me how to do a bowel routine properly, the bitch tore me a new one. Literally.

Fortunately, even though the nurses were a mix of good and terrible, my roommate was a really nice guy. On his closet door, someone had taped a picture of him on a dirt bike. So, right away, I knew I was going to like him. Jason was ten years younger than me, had his own construction business, and was engaged to be married. I liked his sense of humour and felt like we had a lot in common and could become friends.

The big difference between us was that Jason was quadriplegic. He dove into a friend's pool and hit his chin on the bottom, breaking his neck. As a result, he could only move his head and had a limited ability to move his arms. I saw him struggling with the many things I still took for granted, and I was humbled.

I don't think Jason knew this, but he became one of my biggest sources of motivation. Seeing how my accident could have been much worse, I felt compelled to stay positive and grateful for what I could still do. Feeding myself, using the bathroom, getting out of bed on my own (so long as the fucking nursing staff didn't move my chair away from the bed while I was sleeping), getting dressed, and wheeling myself around the hospital. I considered myself lucky. In fact, I tried to be careful not to complain about my challenges to Jason. I assumed he would rather be para than quad any day. From his perspective, I bet he thought I had it easy. From his perspective, I couldn't argue. I was learning quickly that everyone's unique challenges are relative.

And writing about that reality reminds me of an interesting thing I noticed at Lyndhurst. There's a pissing match based on the level of injury that happens whenever you meet someone new in a wheelchair.

The conversations seem to go like this… "What's your name, how'd you get injured, what's your level of injury, are you complete (total paralysis) or incomplete (some signals might be getting through the spinal cord)?" In short order, there is a determination of who has it worse based on the level and severity of your spinal cord injury, and conversely, it is understood who got off "easy," or at least "easier."

I suppose I shouldn't have been surprised that even when it came to a spinal cord injury, that people would make judgements based on one's injury level, just like they do with how you look or what you drive. I'd have to try and not do that myself.

Many of my days in Lyndhurst were incredibly sad. I could get out of my bed on my own, but now I felt like a prisoner in a correctional institution being punished for my impulsiveness and bad luck. A month before, I was looking forward to our upcoming trip to Hawaii. Now, I was held hostage in this hospital, requiring help from everyone around me.

When I was alone or with my closest family, the tears would come. I was grieving what I had lost and growing impatient to be back home with my girls. Sabrina and I parented well together, and with me in the hospital unable to hold up my part of the deal, I felt bad for her and myself. I wanted to be home to wake the girls up in the morning and get them dressed for the day. To feed them a meal and roll around on the playroom floor with them. I missed showing them how to build Lego houses and forts out of sticks, cardboard boxes, and blankets. I wanted my daddy time and knew that I was missing out. I wanted to read them their bedtime stories and find the mouse in *Goodnight Moon*. I wanted to be home.

The only good thing about those tears was that they pushed me to get stronger and to get home as quickly as I could. I focused my mind and all my energy on getting a little stronger every day.

The best days at rehab were when Sabrina came to visit in the afternoon, brought dinner from home and stayed until my bedtime. Our friends gave us DVDs of *24* and *Prison Break,* so we snuggled on my bed and watched a few episodes each visit before Sabrina had to get back home to Chloe and Zara. Our moms took turns taking care of the girls so we could have this time together.

It was a busy time for Sabrina. Overseeing a major, unplanned renovation to accommodate me so I could return to an accessible home was no small feat. She often brought samples of building materials and paint chips so we could choose together. Things happened very quickly, and there were many decisions to be made. It wasn't uncommon for me to be in the middle of physiotherapy and between reps of some exercise when my phone rang. I would stop, take the call, and problem-solve some surprise challenge that needed an answer.

It was crazy. It was exciting. We were moving forward at a hundred miles per hour to get our world back in order. We refused to sit and stew—to feel sorry for ourselves. We had to move forward.

One evening was even better than most because Sabrina brought Chloe and Zara for dinner and a visit. The girls were taking it all in stride: me being in the hospital and not home, combined with all the visitors, flowers, and drama that I can imagine took place at home. Appreciating that our two little girls were still under five years of age, I was impressed with just how well they adapted to change.

I knew when I broke my back, mine wasn't the only life that was turned upside down. So Sabrina and I tried extra hard to make everything seem as normal and as comfortable as possible when we were all together. That evening was special because we were having a meal together again as a family like we would at home. While Sabrina heated and served the dinner, I got busy colouring some pictures with the girls.

Colouring was a great craft to do with the girls because quite often, while we were all working on our pages, the girls would start a conversation or ask a question. Essentially, they were sharing what was on their minds.

Out of the blue, Zara started telling me that I was going to be okay. I put down my crayons and grabbed my phone to record what she wanted to share with me. In her sweet, squeaky voice, she carefully explained that Allah would come and fix my back. Apparently, she'd been talking with Sabrina's mom, who told the girls about Allah and his ability to work miracles. Sabrina and I didn't practice a religion with the girls, so this was a bit of a surprise. Zara shared with me that Allah was sneaky—you couldn't see him, but with scissors and glue, he'd fix my back so that I could walk again. I was fascinated and showed Zara my appreciation and excitement for this news, but I asked her what if Allah couldn't fix my back. Would that be okay? I tried to assure her it was not all bad and that if I was in a wheelchair, I could give her rides on my lap. After much thought (for a 2 ¾-year-old), she told me that it would be fine either way. My heart melted.

After dinner, I tried to engage the girls in a fun game and suggested we play tag in the Lyndhurst foyer. At first, when I tried to catch them, it was impossible. I was too weak, the chair was too heavy, and they were way too fast. We switched, and Chloe would try to catch me. I got a head start and wheeled away as fast as I could. I thought I was doing well, but within no time at all, my chair came to a screeching halt as Chloe grabbed the handles on the back of my chair and stopped me cold. Without any abdominals to hold me up, I fell at the waist and almost tumbled out of my chair.

"New rule: no knocking Daddy out of his chair," I proclaimed.

After our little game of tag and cleaning up the dishes and colouring, I kissed the girls goodnight, and they all headed back home. It was a lovely and memorable visit. But as I wheeled towards the elevators to go to my room, I started crying again. Being separated from my girls was unbearable, and this feeling of isolation made me feel like I was being punished, yet again, with little control over anything important. I was mad at myself for going on that stupid mountain bike ride, for making such an impulsive and immature decision, for being unlucky. I wiped my tears before returning to my room, jumped on the computer, and poured over my blog until it was time to sleep. Another day done.

Winter came early in 2008, and the Don Valley transformed into a majestic snowscape. My room looked out onto the valley, and I could see people from the neighbourhood out running and walking their dogs. It was such a difficult thing to see, knowing that I'd never again have the freedom to put on a pair of shoes and go for a run. It was a brutal way to start the day, but after I had my little cry, I tried to focus my mind on my getting stronger and going home.

I had a lot of visitors at Lyndhurst, which was wonderful. My family and friends, colleagues, and even a few surprises. It was interesting to me how my accident brought people in from the sidelines of my life. Of course, there were many people I expected to visit, and they didn't disappoint. But I was pleasantly surprised by the number of friends, acquaintances and colleagues that showed up to see how I was doing, who I didn't expect would visit. All these characters created the light of my story, and I could never thank all of them enough for their enduring support.

My physiotherapist, Jamie, was the best part of rehab. He pushed me to become stronger and was quick to recognize and leverage the fact that I like to be challenged. I asked him and the other staff about how I might get involved in parasports. Physical activity had been so important to me, especially that year. And I knew that I must continue to be active if I was going to continue to have a full and rewarding life. Sharing my interest in learning more about parasports with everyone I spoke to at Lyndhurst, I was repeatedly asked if I'd met Rich yet.

Rich was the same age as me, but he broke his back when he was 21 years old in a motorcycle accident on the Garden City Skyway, travelling from St Catherine's to Niagara Falls. A truck with a backhoe on a trailer was stopped on the bridge, and when the car travelling in front of Rich swerved out of the way at the last second, Rich didn't see it in time and ran into the backhoe. He broke one bone in his body...his back. At T4, his injury level was higher than mine (let's get that out of the way).

An avid skier and athlete before the accident, Rich threw himself into wheelchair sports after being injured. An innovator as well, Rich represented Canada in three different sports: rowing, tennis, and alpine skiing. He was also accomplished in road racing (wheelchair and handcycling), triathlons, kayaking and scuba diving. In addition to his athletic achievements, Rich earned a B.A. from Brock University and became the first Honour's post-graduate in Therapeutic Recreation in Ontario with a disability. I connected with Rich through email, and Sabrina and I scheduled to meet with him the next day.

We grabbed a small meditation room in Lyndhurst so we could have a little quiet and privacy. I suspected if we met out in the open, every person passing by would want to stop and chat with Rich. My first impression of him was that he could easily be my cousin, if not a brother. Blond with blue eyes, if his last name didn't give away that he's Dutch, his appearance certainly did. Rich was positive, kind, and happy, quick to say something funny to keep the atmosphere light while also being sensitive to the fact that Sabrina and I were still new to this world and likely still a little in shock.

He started by sharing his story with us. He talked about his accident and what came after. You could tell he had told his story many times as he delivered it effortlessly. Throughout our conversation, he shared recommendations of things or strategies that I'd likely find helpful. I took every word to heart and tried to remember it all.

One of the first things Rich asked me was if I was someone who could lower their expectations and compromise. It was a straightforward way of thinking about it. He told me that in his experience, people who could lower their expectations and compromise to any situation adjusted better to life with a spinal cord injury. Those who couldn't, didn't.

While I instinctively knew that some people would disagree with this notion, thinking that, by definition, if you compromise, you never get 100% of what you truly wanted. And, therefore, you would never be as happy as you could possibly be. I also knew that I didn't have this luxury, nor would letting myself contemplate taking that stance do me any good. To insist on things being exactly like they were before my accident, like me walking out of the hospital, would not be helpful or healthy. Being the youngest of four children, I knew that compromise in life was necessary. Now that I was paraplegic, I realized even more how important a positive approach to redefining my life was going to be.

Rich had brought a portfolio to our meeting, and he started pulling out some pictures for Sabrina and me to see. He showed me his motorcycle after the accident, in pieces: its front forks separated from the bike; the front wheel somehow wrapped around a piece on the trailer that carried the backhoe. He explained that he had only glanced back to see his friend for a moment before the car he was following swerved to avoid the stopped truck and trailer. He ran straight into it. It was a shocking picture. Rich then pulled out another picture and presented it to us with a big smile. My jaw dropped.

Damn, I thought to myself, *this guy can fly!*

Imagine a snowy mountain slope, set against a bright blue sky, and right in the middle, a guy in a sit-ski, flying through the air, with his arms spread eagle. There's more than 15 feet of air between his sit-ski and the ground. He appears to be flying.

The second thought that ran through my head was that Rich must not be married, as I knew for a fact that Sabrina, while typically very easygoing and trusting, would never approve of me trying something like this.

This picture cemented for me that anything was possible if I wanted it badly enough. I was grateful to learn this lesson so quickly after my injury. I needed to believe that I, too, could accomplish extraordinary things. It was the most valuable lesson I could learn at that time, and it was taught by someone with the credibility to teach it.

I had a million questions for Rich. Things like, how do you travel on a plane? How do you pee in a public toilet? How do you have sex? He was very kind to share with us how he navigated paraplegia, and the sense of relief I gained from meeting with him was palpable. Not to rush things, but I was hoping we'd become friends. A buddy to do some crazy shit with and to make some fun memories would be amazing.

In addition to Rich, there were several other kind and helpful people (in chairs) who helped me navigate challenges on my path to recovery. Spinal Cord Injury Ontario is in the same building as Lyndhurst, and I benefited greatly from the staff there who also shared with me how they adapted to their injuries to lead fulfilling lives. I was grateful to all the people who offered to help, but Rich was truly an exceptional person that just did it. He showed up and delivered, anticipating what you might want to see, discuss or learn. Over time I learned firsthand just how many people he had this impact on, and I considered myself to be one of those fortunate ones.

Rich showed me I could fly and inspired me to chase after what I wanted, regardless of not being able to use my lower body. And while it wasn't likely to happen on a sit-ski, I knew I wanted nothing more than to experience that kind of power for myself. I wanted to make myself, and more importantly, my girls, proud.

Chapter 5
Family, Friends & Strangers

It's a sad fact that most people who have a spinal cord injury (SCI) can't go back to their homes. Most houses aren't accessible, nor can they be easily renovated to accommodate someone in a wheelchair. This makes being paraplegic even more difficult. In addition to losing their mobility, many people with SCIs must deal with the extra stress, costs, and emotional upheaval for their entire family that results from unexpectedly having to find an accessible place to live.

Sabrina and I wanted to stay in our home; we just had to problem-solve how.

We started our quest to make our home accessible by reaching out to our neighbours, Emma and Sandy, the ones with whom we ran the Oakville half-marathon. They lived two doors down from us, and as they grew up in Oakville, I had a suspicion that Sandy might know how to get a building permit quickly. It turned out that I was wrong about the permit knowledge. But ever the resourceful couple, they immediately introduced themselves to our other neighbours, John and Marcia, who lived further down the street. John and Marcia were architects. Emma and Sandy shared what happened to me and our hope that we'd be able to find a way to stay in our home.

John and Marcia had heard about my accident on the news but didn't realize it was someone who lived just a few houses away. John's firm specialized in designing commercial institutions, like hospitals, but they were moved by my story and wanted to help if they could.

The next evening, John and Marcia came over to meet Sabrina and Amir and to look at our home. After a quick walk through the house, they thought that an elevator could be installed using one of the spaces in the garage. Doing so would allow me a way into our home from the outside and then provide access into the basement, the main floor foyer, and the upstairs hallway. We'd need to reconfigure three of the upstairs bedrooms to make it work, but it was possible.

Sabrina gave me regular updates on John's progress. Going above and beyond, John took some holidays from work to focus on our project. He met with an elevator company to figure out options and specifications and spent half a day at Oakville's Town Hall, learning the ins and outs of getting this residential building permit.

As October was coming to an end, John called Sabrina and asked her to come to the Town Hall—with the girls. He'd done everything required to get the permit and felt that if the good folks at the planning department met the girls, they'd be compelled to provide the permit today. He was right. We got the building permit! The renovations could now begin.

John was a very busy man, so for him to make time to help out a young family down the street that he didn't previously know touched our hearts deeply. In addition to his thoughtfulness, John wouldn't accept any form of payment other than our gratitude. John and Marcia's generosity set the stage for what would become an amazing home renovation completed in a short amount of time, thanks to the help of many friends, family members, and strangers.

What's Next

In conversation with one of my therapists, I was told that it's quite common for individuals who suffer a spinal cord injury to immediately deny the reality of their accident and consequently refuse to take action to make their world accessible. They'll often say, "I'll leave the hospital when I can walk out of here."

Sabrina and I were the total opposite. Having acknowledged that my injury was permanent, we were determined to get me back into our home as quickly as possible, doing whatever was necessary to make our home as accessible as we could, based on what we knew and what we could quickly learn. Being able to stay in our home and our neighbourhood was a blessing. With neighbours like Emma and Sandy, and John and Marcia, we felt lucky to be the recipients of so much kindness.

My neighbours were the closest people to me geographically, but of course, in terms of relationships, no one is closer than family. From the moment my family learned about my injury, they began mobilizing to help my girls and me through this.

I grew up the youngest of four kids, separated by seven years, with two older brothers, Jim and Rick, followed by my sister, Doralyn. Even though we didn't see each other often, there has always been a lot of love among us. My father was a contractor, building everything from homes to the kind of retail stores you'll find in your neighbourhood mall. From the age of 13 until I got married and moved away, I enjoyed learning from and working with my dad and my brother, Rick, who took over the family business when my dad passed away in 2002.

From the ICU onward, my siblings had been by my side (literally and emotionally). While I focused on healing from my injuries, Rick strategized with Sabrina, Amir, and my neighbour John on how to make our home accessible. Within days of John and Marcia's first visit, Rick called me up and shared with me that he was going to lead the home renovation. It wasn't even a question, such as "Would you like me to do this?" It was a statement. He had chatted with Jim and my many cousins (a surprising number who are also tradesmen) and reassured me that I had nothing to worry about; it was all going to be taken care of. I was speechless and so grateful. Even though I was 37 years old, moments like this reminded me of that safe, protective feeling you got as a child when your older siblings ensured that nothing and no one would harm you.

In rehab, I worked hard to build my strength and independence—progress was slow going, but it was progress. Fortunately, as November came to an end, I was given permission to go home for a night or two on the weekends.

My first trip home for a night involved stopping at a dance studio in Milton, a growing town north of Oakville, where Sabrina had organized Chloe's fifth birthday party. Everyone was happy to see me out, and I was thrilled to be able to stop in, but it didn't take long for me to be exhausted and overwhelmed by all the excitement and effort required to be there. I did my best to help Chloe celebrate. But soon after cake was served, I excused myself and had someone take me home so I could lay down.

The guest bed was moved into our dining room, so I didn't need to go upstairs. At home, it was the first time I'd been back since that Sunday morning of my accident. The house looked a little chaotic. But with two little ones and me in the hospital, this is how I should have expected it to look. It felt so good to be home. I scanned my living room, quickly assessing the couch and chairs to determine if they were an option for me this day. I wanted to transfer to one of them and relax, but I was worried I might not have the strength to successfully make it out and back into my wheelchair again if I went for it. I was also worried about having an accident on our furniture, as I was still trying to learn how to manage my bladder and bowels. Rather than risk a setback, I settled on transferring to the bed, but not before grabbing the blueprints for the elevator and renovation that I saw rolled up on the kitchen counter.

It was exciting to read the blueprints and see what John had planned for our home. It all looked so professional and official, and I was pumped at knowing that on Monday, the work could start. Installing an elevator in an existing home was no small task. As I looked at the space where the elevator shaft was destined to go, I realized that a lot had to be done to prepare our home for this reno. Essentially, the house was going to be ripped open from the basement to the upstairs floor, but before that could happen, the furniture and everything else in the impacted rooms needed to be removed or, at least, set aside and covered. Even though it was getting late that Saturday night, I sent out an email to friends asking for help in the morning.

It felt great to wake up in my own home, and after a nice breakfast, we started welcoming friends in. By nine o'clock, eleven friends had already arrived. They were ready to move, stack, and cover all the furniture from the various rooms into the great room. Across the opening to the kitchen from the great room, they taped a curtain of clear poly in the hopes of keeping some of the dust out of the kitchen. With bodies and furniture racing around in every direction, it was amazing to see so much happen so quickly. Taking apart the beds and stacking the furniture was stunning to see. And it felt so wonderful to receive so much help, especially on such short notice. Chloe and Zara were in awe, too, as this was a lot of commotion and excitement for a Sunday morning.

With me back in rehab the following week, Sabrina came for a mid-week visit. She shared with me how Chloe was trying to piece together what was happening in their lives with all of the people coming and going and having to move into her grandmother's home while the renovation happened.

Chloe asked Sabrina: "So because Daddy has helped all of these friends in the past, now that Daddy is hurt, they're all coming to help him?" Sabrina nodded and said, "Yes." Chloe had got it exactly right.

After my first visit home on the weekend, I began going to my mother-in-law's with the girls. It was a beautiful loft-bungalow home with lots of room for me to wheel around and everything I needed on the main floor. Honestly, though, anything was better than the hospital, especially if I could be with my girls.

We spent our Saturday morning sleeping in, playing games and colouring, as well as making lists of things we needed to pick up at Home Depot and specialty shops in the afternoon. This was all prep for Sunday, when we'd join a crew of five to fifteen friends, family and strangers, who showed up to work on our home.

The renovation was extensive and required concrete work and framing, drywall, and trim. We were replacing most of the existing doors with much wider three-foot ones that made it easier for me to get through in my wheelchair, replacing all the carpet with hardwood and redoing our ensuite bathroom, and finishing the basement.

It was a big job, but everyone working on it did so with a smile on their face and a spring in their step. There was a good vibe of helping us out, and often that energy was stoked by the fact that each day became a little family-and-friends reunion of sorts. In addition to my brothers being there, my cousins and uncles also came out to lend a hand, as did lots of friends and colleagues from work, some even spending their weekends to accelerate the progress on our reno.

I've always had a real affection for my cousins. Some of my fondest memories of growing up involved doing fun (and at times dangerous) things with them. With both my parents being one of nine siblings, I have over 50 first cousins. Most are in the London, Ontario, area. Growing up, my friends loved to joke that it was impossible for me to leave my house and not run into a cousin.

I suppose they were right, especially when I think back to that time a group of high school friends and I ran into my cousin Jacquie unexpectedly while hanging out in Toronto for a day. And then it even happened on a different continent when I was backpacking through Europe after high school and met my cousin, Yvonne, for the first time. I was passing through a train station in Holland when I heard someone yelling, "Cousin! Cousin!" She saw my Canadian flag on my backpack, and I looked like I could be family, so she took a chance. What a crazy experience that was. I guess I did have cousins everywhere.

Extended family is special. There's something unique about everyone, but we all share our history and core values. Seeing so many come to aid in my recovery was a little overwhelming but in a good way.

Adding to those generously giving their time to help us was my brother Jim's friend, who was also named Jim. Jim is an electrician whom I'd never met before. Upon hearing my story and situation, Jim and his crew (who live and work over an hour away) started driving to Oakville to complete all the electrical work required for the reno. When I tried to pay Jim, he would only let me pay for the materials they used. I was a little dumbfounded. So much generosity from people I didn't know. And, when the renos were done, even my sister and aunts would get in on the action, coming to Oakville to clean our home so I could return to a renovated and show-worthy home. I felt so lucky.

It was a powerful feeling to have family, friends, and strangers rallying to support me in a time of need. And even though I was still in rehab, I felt involved in the renovation by helping to make decisions with Sabrina and Rick, as well as by being on site in the house on Sundays.

December was a bit of a blur, but as Christmas approached, I informed the hospital that I was going home for a week. I don't think the nurses and doctors particularly liked my idea, but I didn't care. The girls and I stayed at my mother-in-law's home and had the place to ourselves, as she and her husband went away on a cruise. Having so much time with my girls and being able to spend every day helping (or overseeing) with the reno at our home was exactly what I needed. By this time, even though the elevator wasn't finished, I could get to all the floors of my home. Fortunately for me, everyone helping was kind and open to my suggestions and requests with regards to the renovation. Even though it was difficult, at best, for a newbie like me to navigate a wheelchair around a construction site with debris, tools, supplies, and takeout scattered everywhere, it was incredibly satisfying to be able to get to every room in my home again and see the progress firsthand. My home. I knew how lucky I was to be able to say this. To still have it.

Looking back, it's no surprise Sundays became my favourite day of the week. I knew my family and friends, and friends of friends, would be coming to help in the renovation, which in turn would allow me to come home for good. As enjoyable as these Sundays were, though, they weren't without tears and heartache as I was forced to start acknowledging what I'd lost when I broke my back. Even before I started officially doing construction at the age of thirteen, I had grown up admiring my dad and brother and loved to build things. As a kid, my favourite pastime was Legos. And when I was old enough to swing a hammer and later to use small power tools to fashion something out of scraps that were left around the house, I would. Having worked for my dad's business for so many years, I couldn't imagine how many sheets of drywall I've installed, cabinets I crafted, or doors that I've hung and trimmed; the number would be significant. Construction and fine woodworking were skills that I honed over many years and was very proud to have.

When we moved into our home before Chloe was born, I used half of the basement to build myself a dream workshop. With built-in dust collection to all the machines, cabinets, and shelves for storage, and tall counters to work on, this was my home inside my home. A place where I could lose myself and express my creative side. A place in my house that I now wondered if I'd ever be able to fully enjoy again, being in a wheelchair. My home was full of beautiful things I built and that would last forever, but I made those when I could walk. *How the hell can I do anything now?* I asked myself. All this work on our home needed to be done. I wanted to physically do it, but I couldn't. I felt like a spectator being forced to watch friends work on my home while I was stuck in my chair. It hurt badly.

So many things got me in a knot as I tried hard not to have a total emotional meltdown. They could be stupid things too. Like when a friend insisted on cutting a piece of drywall bigger than I suggested and then was surprised when it broke while screwing it to the wall. I gave him the dimensions to purposely cut it a little smaller than the opening it needed to fit into, but he wanted it to be the exact same size as the opening. I couldn't be rude and insist on doing it my way, as he was there on his Sunday helping me renovate my home. I had to be grateful and not in any way critical. But if only I could have grabbed the knife, climbed the ladder, and done this myself, it would have been done right the first time. And I would have been the one responsible for it.

Damn! Watching was so much harder than doing. It was a unique torture specific to me, and it was only drywall. I wasn't sure how I was going to be able to accept my new limitations beyond the home reno. I snuck away to another room to have a cry in private.

I still loved Sundays, but having to accept that there were things I couldn't do anymore was crushing. Intellectually, I tried to deconstruct what was going on in my gut and my brain in hopes that a textbook rationalization might make understanding and accepting it easier. My brain went to what I knew, which was sociology – the focus of my undergrad and graduate degrees. I thought about the concept of identity. I knew my injury was forcing me to redefine my old identity with something new.

But I liked who I was. I was okay with so much of what I could do physically being wrapped up in my core identity of who I was.

That was my brand; that was ME. If I had to change, I knew I would fight to make sure that I was the one who defined my new identity. There was no way I was going to let my identity become that of a helpless person using a wheelchair, yet when I looked in the mirror, that is exactly what I saw. Thinking about what Rich said to me, maybe I could find a compromise. Maybe I could convince myself and those around me to see me as a recovering husband, dad and friend, for the immediate future. I'd work on rebuilding my brand into something that I could be proud of later on.

On another Sunday afternoon, in January, most of my friends had gone home for the day when I decided I would have a go at sweeping the bathroom floor by myself. Our original ensuite with a glass shower and claw-foot tub were totally inaccessible for me in the wheelchair, so it had to be gutted. With the big stuff disposed of, the bathroom floor was still a mess from the demolition and the beginning of the repair. I grabbed a broom and a putty knife and began to scrape and clean the floor.

The last thing I expected was a lesson in science, but that's what I got. For every action—in this case, pushing a broom or scraping the floor—there was an equal and opposite reaction. Without the brakes applied, my chair moved away from the very thing I was trying to work on. When I pushed the broom away, I wheeled backwards away from the dirt. When I swept towards myself, I pulled my wheelchair over the dirt. Newton's Third Law of Motion didn't give a shit that I was exhausted, frustrated, and in pain.

Refusing to give up, I figured out how to maneuver myself into just the right position, lock the brakes on the chair, sweep a few feet of floor, and then repeat the process. Just moving the broom was so difficult, but the greater challenge was bending over in my chair to scoop up the debris and put it into the small box I was using to collect the garbage while being careful not to lean so far forward that I would fall out of my chair. With no working abs, I used one hand to hold onto my chair while I held myself in the sitting position and tried my best not to spill all of the debris from the dustpan so I could get it into the box. I was dumbfounded that something so simple before my accident could be so frustratingly difficult now. It took me an hour just to sweep this 10x10 room. By the end, I was exhausted and sad but tried to find some sense of accomplishment in a task as trivial as sweeping a room.

This was my rehab. I needed to relearn how to do everything physical, but from my wheelchair. Fortunately, I was gifted with being stubborn and determined.

At the end of the day, thinking about my Sunday, I revisited and reconfirmed how I was going to respond to breaking my back. In terms of things that I was able to do, I decided I would just start at the bottom again, like my little girls. I'd conquer all the basics and then get into the more difficult things as I gained my strength. I'd figure it out and do it, even though it wouldn't be easy. The last thing I was going to do was just watch while others worked on my home. I was going to do what little things I could to contribute. If I was being forced to redefine my identity, this is where I was going to start.

I knew full well that my old life was gone, even though I'd often disregard that awareness and throw myself into things that others thought I couldn't or shouldn't do. Over the years before my accident, I had put a lot of work and love into our house. I'd personally fashioned some of the finer pieces of cabinetry and some built-ins, a couple of the beds, some mirrors and wall boxes for Chloe's bedroom. During 2005, I had invested at least four weeks of full-time work (including holidays from the office) into building and finishing a mission-style dresser. It was a solid quarter-sawn white oak beast, 40 inches high by 90 inches wide with ten drawers, all grain-matched and dovetailed. It was heavier than you could imagine, and it was almost perfect. It was truly a one-of-a-kind piece, and I had designed and crafted it by myself.

After my accident, on one of the Sundays at our house, I was floored to find the dresser covered in a mess of dust, tools, and coffee cups. A mini breakdown ensued. This was the finest piece of furniture I had ever built in my life, and I felt like it was being treated like a scrap workbench in the furnace room. The faces of the drawers had been scratched by the tools and construction materials leaned against them. There was even a big-ass crowbar laying directly on the wooden top! For a moment, I was devastated that no one seemed to think about just how precious this furniture could be to me. This was the finest work of cabinetry I had ever completed and something I'd never be able to build again on my own, and it was being damaged because of simple carelessness.

Of course, no one intentionally meant to do any harm to me or my furniture. They were there giving up their free time to help me, so I'd never say anything negative. But man, I never expected Rich's advice about learning to compromise to appear in such a random way. I knew there were some things I'd need to learn to let go of and some things that I couldn't control or do on my own anymore. Perfection probably shouldn't be the yardstick to measure success anymore, and I'd have to be okay with that. But it was going to be so difficult.

The feeling that I had lost my trade, the ability to complete fine woodworking with the precision and speed that I used to—skills I had honed for over 25 years—was extremely difficult. I knew I was lucky that this wasn't my career, but it was still something that generated a lot of personal pride and something I still wanted to be able to do. In time, I accepted the reality that I'd find a way to be almost as good as I was, and it would be okay if I never liked that particular compromise. This was my life, and I had to deal with it.

It was apparent that I had more grieving to do. Sabrina came and consoled me, and she helped me clean off and protect the dresser so that more damage was not likely to happen. But a couple of layers of cardboard and painter's tape could only do so much. Similar to how my house was being adapted to make it livable for me, I needed to work on my mind and start making those changes that would allow me to let go of things that I couldn't control or were not fundamentally important and just find a way to move on.

I had always enjoyed helping others, and I definitely preferred to be that guy as opposed to being the one asking for help. Unfortunately, a spinal cord injury demands that you open yourself up to the assistance of others. This was a tough lesson for someone like me, and it was certainly not something I was comfortable learning to do.

One evening, after my cousin Paul finished drywalling the elevator shaft, I shared with him my frustrations. And he, in turn, shared his thoughts, which were that people really enjoyed helping me out and that it was good for me to let them. Doing so made them feel good. This wasn't rocket science, but I acknowledged that it was solid advice to remember. For my family and friends, and the new friends I meet along the way, helping me could be a way for them to process what has happened and strengthen our friendships and shared community. I had to broaden my perspective to see this, but as time passed, this understanding helped me learn to be more comfortable accepting help from others.

And if all this help from friends and family wasn't already at times overwhelming, things got taken to the next level when their friends came out to help as well. People who were essentially strangers to me gave up their Sundays to pitch in on the renovation. I hoped that all the good deeds I had done before the accident had accrued me some credit in the karma bank because I certainly was making a lot of withdrawals.

Regardless of all the mental and physical challenges I had, I took great comfort in knowing that I wasn't alone. If a person were to measure his wealth by the number and quality of his friends and family, then I was very wealthy indeed. In some ways, my accident was turning out to be a clarifying experience. How people responded to me in my time of need proved the importance of family, friends, and strangers. On a daily basis, I was touched by the goodwill and kind deeds of so many who stepped up and showed me their true character. This included new people entering our lives, who I felt were likely to become some of the best friends we would ever have.

Chapter 6

Pushing Hard – Going Nowhere

I've never believed that feeling sorry for oneself does anyone any good. So I didn't wallow in self-pity or spend any time questioning why it was me who broke his back even though I had friends who did crazier shit all the time. All my energy was focused on getting the hell out of rehab and on with my life. I knew if I wanted my life back quickly, I needed to learn everything I could about my injury. And, more importantly, how others in my situation adapted.

Shortly after leaving rehab and returning home, it came to my attention that some people were concerned I hadn't grieved enough for my loss. This came as a bit of a surprise. Were people wanting me to be unproductive and sad to see that I was grieving what I lost? And how long would be enough time for them to feel like I had grieved properly? These questions (and people) just upset me. Didn't they know that's not my thing? I could accept that my response to my accident might not be textbook for someone dealing with a catastrophic injury, but I tried not to care what they thought.

My accident was kind of like those times in life when you literally fall down and immediately jump back up, and before you've even done an inventory of your health, you proclaim that: "I'm good, I'm okay, nothing to see here." That's how I responded to breaking my back.

First, let me ensure that my home and girls are sorted out and okay, then let me prove to myself that I can still do enough with just my arms to make life productive and rewarding, and to make my girls proud, and then, once all that's taken care of, I'll get to the messy stuff of my emotions and grieving. If you couldn't see the value in my approach, then I really didn't need to hear your opinion.

When I broke my back, the doctors in rehab were required to notify the Ministry of Transportation. Not long after, I received a letter from the Ministry indicating that in order for me to keep my driver's license, I'd have to recertify by passing a driving test. From the moment my chest tube was removed, and I wasn't preoccupied with dying from my lungs collapsing or contracting pneumonia, I began the process of learning everything I could about driving with just my upper body.

In rehab, the patients were encouraged to have three goals to work towards. The intention was to provide patients with focus and goals that moved them closer to being able to return home. This exercise was easy for me, as I had my goals established before they even told me of this protocol. Getting my driver's license was my first goal. The second was to be fitted for as many sports chairs as possible. And the third was to learn more wheelchair skills than anyone else who had left rehab so that when I was out in the real world, I'd be able to navigate any obstacle on my own or direct others on how to help me.

I was able to start working on the driver's license while still in rehab. I learned from my physiotherapist (PT), Jamie, that the first thing I needed to do was connect with a special clinic twenty minutes away from Lyndhurst, where an occupational therapist (OT) would assess my strength, vision, balance, coordination, and movement.

Once that was completed, they'd take me in an adapted vehicle for a test drive to see how I could manage.

There was a car in rehab fitted with hand controls that Jamie introduced me to during one of my PT sessions. As we made our way over to the car, Rich wheeled by and saw what we were up to and stopped to share his experiences and advice. He showed me how he transfers into the car and disassembles his chair to bring it into the car as well. He made it look so easy.

As for the hand controls, they were surprisingly simple. Basically, there is one lever controlled with your left hand and mounted under the steering wheel with a bracket. It's on a pivot and connected to two rods. One rod connects to the accelerator so that when you pull the lever towards you, the vehicle is given gas. The other rod is connected to the brake pedal so that pushing the lever away from you applies the brake. I was eager to try it out for myself for real.

A week later, at my scheduled driving assessment in North Toronto, I had my chance. The physical tests were fine and must have gone well enough, as following the assessment, they asked me if I was ready to try driving in their minivan equipped with hand controls. The main OT that I had been working with sat in one of the back seats. Her colleague, whom I assumed to be the driving instructor guy, sat in the passenger seat and explained to me how everything worked. Stop, go, turn, turn, stop… it was easy, and I was thrilled to get on with it. Funny enough, this experience reminded me of the first time I ever drove a car. I felt like I was sixteen again and one step closer to gaining my freedom.

Out on the road amidst traffic, I must have been doing a good job because the OT asked me if I'd ever done this before. "No," I told him. It was just easy. Maybe using my hands to drive was instinctive to me because I'd ridden so many motorcycles throughout my life. It just felt natural. I loved driving, so I was happy to be in control of a vehicle again. I wished they would just give me my license back right away after doing a good job in their minivan. Unfortunately, though, it was not that easy. And while I understood why, I didn't like it.

Following our drive around the neighbourhood, I asked the assessment administrator how many lessons I'd have to take before I could do my driving test. She told me that most people required ten hours of lessons using hand controls for the actions to become second nature and dependable. Apparently, many people learn how to drive with hand controls reasonably quickly. But when surprised in an emergency, their instinct to brake with their feet takes over, and they crash into something or someone.

I had to take her word for it that most people required ten hours of lessons. But at $175 an hour and having just been told that I did great on my first outing, there was no way I was doing all ten lessons. I asked her what the fewest number of lessons was that anyone had ever taken to prepare for and pass the driver's test. She told me four. "Okay," I said. I could agree to four lessons, but that was it.

While I was in Hamilton General Hospital just days after breaking my back, I started researching new cars online. At the time of my accident, my car was a six-speed manual transmission Infiniti that required the use of my feet for not only the gas and brake pedals but also for the clutch pedal. In doing research, I discovered some fancy racing controls that could allow you to drive a standard transmission car with only your hands, but they were complicated and expensive. On top of that complexity, my car was a four-door that I was told would be difficult to transfer my 6'2" body into from a wheelchair. And it would be even more difficult to fold up my wheelchair and lift it over me onto the passenger seat so I could be truly independent.

Around Lyndhurst, I asked everyone in wheelchairs what kind of cars they drove, along with the benefits and disadvantages of each type. Most paraplegics recommended coupes—good-looking cars with one wide door on each side that allowed more space for getting you and your chair in and out.

One or two people recommended an adapted minivan for its practicality. Basically, you can wheel up a ramp that comes out of the side opening of the minivan. But this screamed "medical device" to me, and that would ultimately suck the joy out of the driving experience. So I kindly told them that while I appreciated the recommendation, I wasn't ready to swallow that life change just yet. Yes, I couldn't walk anymore, but no, I wasn't ready for minivan life. With the search for a speedy coupe underway, I had a great project to focus my mind on.

On the trip home for Christmas and New Years, my friends and I stopped and checked out some new cars in the dealership to see how easily I could get in and out and where my chair could go if I had all of my girls with me in the car. It was fun to figure all this out, even with so much other stuff going on.

January was cold and snowy, with the weather just adding to my difficulty of navigating life from a wheelchair. After an extended stay in Oakville over Christmas and New Years, I came back to rehab and informed the staff and administration that I was ready to go home for good. I broke my back on October 5th, so I was happy to be heading back home after just three months in hospital and rehab. Our house wouldn't be finished for a few more weeks, but the elevator was working well enough, and we could sleep in our guest bedroom for a few days while our primary bedroom and bath were being finished. It was great to be back home.

A week or two after moving home, it was new car day. I had decided on a new Infiniti G37s in pearl white with automatic and paddle-controlled Tiptronic transmission. And I was excited: the car was in. My excitement was somewhat tempered by the reality of buying a car but not being the person driving it off the lot. My good friend had volunteered to be my legs for the day, so we made the best of it. He loved speed too, so in good form, the first thing he did in my new car was turn off the traction control. Lighting up the tires and peeling out of the dealership had us smiling and giggling like teenage boys. This car would work just fine.

Our first stop was to another friend's tire shop for winter rims and tires, followed by dropping it off at a local accessibility shop to have a guy install the hand controls. In a few days, Sabrina would bring me to pick it up, and I'd be able to drive it home. I couldn't wait.

When it came to living without the use of my lower body, not every solution was as simple as buying a new car with hand controls. I considered myself to be a fixer, a problem-solver, and all my life, I've excelled at doing just that. But the next challenge might just be my biggest problem yet and would likely test my insistence on fixing everything quickly. I wanted to make love to my beautiful wife.

Married for 12 and a half years, Sabrina and I had a healthy marriage, both emotionally and physically. Not that I discussed this with my friends, but I assumed that for a younger couple with two kids under the age of five, our sex life was at least average, if not a little better.

When I sustained a spinal cord injury, in addition to losing my mobility, I also lost the ability to get an erection. To say it's awkward to write about something so private is an understatement. But if I am to be truly open and honest about the impacts of an SCI, it's important to include the more difficult and uncomfortable challenges that an SCI often forces a person and their partner to face.

Our culture, and especially my gender, is preoccupied, if not obsessed, with physical power. Getting an erection and being able to please your partner is for many an unspoken benchmark for what it means to "be a man." While I was far less concerned with how others assessed manhood, it was important to me that I could still do my part to keep our marriage happy. I was never consumed with this, but it did weigh on my mind.

The doctors in rehab, knowing that my injury was T11/T12, but paralysis was T7, were quick to tell me that I may never get an erection again. To them, it was a clinical reality, and they didn't seem at all empathetic as my eyes welled with tears at hearing this news. Of the three or four ideas they had, the easiest and most convenient thing to try involved medications like Viagra and Cialis. Even though I knew I wouldn't be able to feel it, I'd be happy if the medication could give me something that could work. Even though it was never going to be the same, hopefully we could figure out some new things to keep the physical intimacy in our relationship strong. Now that we were in our home again, I asked Sabrina if we could try.

Sabrina had been following my lead with most decisions since my accident. So when I told her that this was important and I wanted to try and solve it, she was open to trying even though I was sure that she was as tired and stressed as I was.

One evening, when the girls were in bed asleep, I took the little blue pill. In bed, just holding each other felt so wonderful. It had been so long, and I missed this so much. Moving around in bed with just your arms was surprisingly difficult, but we tried to ignore the pauses while I sorted out all my limbs. After around 20 minutes, I hoped that something down below would be building. Unfortunately, there was nothing happening downtown. No response. Nothing.

We hadn't discussed how we'd feel if things didn't work, but of course, I was frustrated and disappointed. I wanted so badly for this to work. The funny thing was, I didn't know how important this was to her. Of course, I could have asked her. But I was afraid that if she told me it was really important, the additional pressure that I was already putting on myself would just make things worse for me. We kissed goodnight, and I turned my body away from her to cry myself to sleep, trying to be as quiet as I could so she wouldn't hear me.

Back at rehab for a checkup, I shared with my doctors my lack of success with the medication. They reassured me that it doesn't always work the first time and suggested that we try again. If it continued to not work, they had some different medications that might have a more positive effect.

The way they talked about having sex was so frustrating. They made it sound easy, like playing some simple game where you just keep taking shots until you hit the target. These caregivers were adults, so I couldn't understand how they didn't seem to appreciate the mental toll that all of this was taking on me. On us.

My marriage with Sabrina was rock solid. Married for over a decade, physical intimacy had always complemented our relationship but never defined it. And with all the other changes in our lives at this time, figuring out sex was just too much. It was way too stressful and disappointing. The cycle of anticipation, effort, and frustration when it didn't happen made me feel terrible about myself. It was one thing if I could never have an orgasm again. I figured that was just one of my punishments for fucking up on my bike. But I still wanted to physically be there for my wife. That continued to be at least as important now as it was before my accident.

After four or five attempts, though, we hit pause on trying to solve this challenge right away. I was hitting a wall, and it was driving me crazy. I couldn't fix it. I hoped that some time would allow me to settle my worries and ease the stress I had started to associate with sex. And for a few months, I thought I was doing well. But then, a road trip with a few friends stirred up my anxiety to a whole new level.

It was summer, and while I valued being able to go outside and play with the girls, I also needed some me time. Specifically, I was off for an overnight outing with some buddies. The first stop was for some dinner and a beer before the fun started. As we went around the table catching up and sharing stories, a recently divorced friend of a friend started recounting the more salacious exploits of his new independence. Without going into too many details—though he did, and they were quite colourful—it involved his affair with some hot, young married woman who was not being satisfied at all by her much older husband. That was all I needed to hear to start spiralling. Thinking of Sabrina, I narrowly avoided having a panic attack right there in the restaurant.

What's Next

I'd lived with my injury for over eight months by this time, and I thought Sabrina and I had gotten through our initial hurdles with physical intimacy. But admittedly, sex was still a sensitive subject for me, and hearing this guy brag about his sex life triggered and intensified my insecurities that I had shelved away. How could I not worry that Sabrina didn't have the same complaints as this woman in buddy's story, and would her commitment to me wane as she felt compelled to find some other guy? These thoughts festered.

Back at home, after my little trip, everything seemed fine, but I was losing sleep over the idea that I wasn't enough for my beautiful wife. It had been a week since my trip, and my fears had only intensified. I decided to reach out to the psychologist at Lyndhurst that I had met with a few times while in rehab. She was wonderful. She understood the challenges of an SCI, and I felt that she really knew the core of who I was and those in my life that were most important to me.

A week later, I was in her office. As I hoped, she was thoughtful and compassionate when I shared my concerns, reassuring me that Sabrina cared about me, that she loved me, and that I didn't need to worry about her looking for another man. I choked back tears as I tried to speak and thanked her for easing my concerns. It was helpful having someone to talk to about this, and I hoped to myself that I could keep these fears of losing my wife at bay. Allowing myself to even think for a minute about a life without my girls was terrifying. I assumed that divorce was common among men who suffered an SCI, but I had to trust that my marriage was secure, that Sabrina and I would continue to be a strong and vibrant couple, despite all that I'd lost—that *we'd* lost.

Sabrina had never given me any reason to worry, but she didn't need to. We often joked that worrying was one of the things that I brought to our relationship. In order not to spiral downwards, even before my accident, I worked hard at reminding myself to stay focused on the right things and not allow myself to get bogged down with made-up worries. Especially when most of the things I was likely anxious about would never actually happen. What I had to do was focus on what I still had and not on what I might lose. I had to always direct my attention towards the things I could do versus the things I couldn't. I had to constantly tell myself that any fear of potentially losing Sabrina wasn't real and that stressing about it was a waste of both time and energy.

Sabrina was a great partner, and I was always amazed that I never heard her complain about my accident and how it impacted her. I knew that the changes to our lives brought about by my injury were not what she signed up for or envisioned when we got married. Even though we all say "for better or worse" in our marriage vows, I don't think most people actually consider what the "worse" side of that contract might entail. I know I certainly didn't.

My buddy, Sabrina, always had my back. She was the only person in my world that I knew would never let me down. Throughout our marriage, our relationship had always been strong. Not once did we have a heated argument. Sure, we disagreed on things, but we never fought. Both of our fathers were prone to heated exchanges (adult tantrums), so we knew firsthand that no good ever came from raising your voice and going off the deep end. I suppose it can be a way to make the person venting feel a little better for a period of time, but that selfishly comes at the expense of everyone else. Instead, if we had a problem, we typically went silent for a short period of time and then thoughtfully talked it through when the time was right.

In terms of what can challenge a marriage, though, a spinal cord injury was unlike anything we had faced before. It was the kind of challenge you never imagined needing to face. Yet there we were, married twelve years with two young daughters. Trying to work our way through the "worse."

Beyond my marriage, one of my greatest fears after breaking my back was the potential of being left behind by my friends—both literally and figuratively.

This is where social media can really hurt a person with a disability. Platforms like Facebook allow us to maintain contact with a broad network of friends, which is great. But when you see everyone living their "best lives" while you're facing a new reality that doesn't seem to include all the things you loved doing, this can mess up your head in a hurry.

For me, something as simple as friends posting pictures of a bike ride could completely ruin my day. Seeing them do all the things that I loved to do but couldn't was beyond difficult. A bike ride, a motorcycle trip, attending a concert, travelling abroad... All these things that were enjoyed in my absence just added to my sadness building below the surface. It was extra difficult when I knew that if I hadn't broken my back, I would have been a big part of the fun. And even if I acknowledge to myself that I might not have joined them on any or all these activities for other reasons, the reality provided little to no comfort. Of course, my friends weren't doing anything wrong. They were living their lives. But why did it have to hurt so badly to see it?

I think it's important to note that, for the most part, friends did invite me to come along for many activities. The problem was that even though there were few things more enjoyable than proving to people that I could do something they thought I couldn't (or shouldn't), saying yes to anything for the first time was always hard to do. I think it boiled down to three main reasons.

First, it was stressful doing anything for the first time as a paraplegic. Even if I spent hours trying to anticipate what might happen during the activity, something new always revealed itself, often some little detail that turned a fun diversion into a complex and worrisome task. Second, it was hard getting beyond the question of "why bother?" It was easy to assume that the thing I wanted to do wasn't going to be as good as it would have been if I could still walk. I didn't want to limit my friends' fun, even though I knew they'd say I wasn't. This fear in my mind was difficult to ignore. And lastly, everything was just so much harder. It's a simple reality that anything you could do with your entire body was going to be many times harder when you were using only your arms. Even though I was good at digging deep to put in the extra effort on top of everything else I had to do to just live, it was exhausting and just easier and safer to decline and stay home.

And it wasn't just about me either. I also worried that whatever we set out to do would prove to be too much for those inviting me, and I'd ultimately be putting them in a difficult situation. Even when I tried to spell it out for them, some of my friends and acquaintances just couldn't comprehend my challenges and concerns. Fortunately, a select few of my very best friends truly didn't care if my presence complicated things. They were better at empathizing and acknowledging my actual challenges, and they were willing to put in the effort to understand my concerns. In fact, I think some even liked the added challenge. These friends quickly found the balance of being attentive to my needs without being overbearing. They were special and did whatever needed to be done to make every outing a success.

On the topic of friends, within the first couple years of my accident, I learned that some people in your life are true friends, but others are just people who happen to share your interests. When I was first hurt, everyone was around and showed their support. But over time, because I couldn't do the activities that were the core of some friendships, we quickly fell out of contact.

It was a fine line between trying to be my old self and adjusting to my new reality. My old life was work hard and play hard. And playing hard often meant drinking hard, going all night, and still being able to function the next day. I was trying to get that back, and there were plenty of beers to be had on renovation Sundays. But, as the months passed and I found opportunities to get properly liquored up, it always ended badly.

In terms of volume and enthusiasm, I could still drink like I did before my accident. The problem was that trying to manage myself as a paraplegic was a totally different ball game. There was no possible way for me to function as I used to when I could walk. Unable to feel my bowel or bladder, the fun usually ended when I noticed I had pissed myself.

Even when I did an IC after every couple of drinks, the nights all too often ended with my pants wet and a chair cushion smelling of urine. Before, going to bed and doing my routine of transferring to the toilet and then the shower was tricky at the best of times, so trying to do this drunk with my balance and strength compromised was a terrible idea. When I was lucky, it all went fine. But way too often, it became a tragic mess, especially when the alcohol loosened my stool, and I shit myself too. These messes further fueled my drunken sadness. Sober, I did a really good job controlling the sadness and grief for what I've lost. But nights of overindulgence ended up becoming a *Why the fuck is this happening to me?* circus of tears and sadness.

Sabrina was always patient with me as I sat on my shower chair, bawling my eyes out. If I was desperate enough to ask, she quietly helped me clean myself, my clothes, and the chair. She could have easily told me that I was a stupid idiot, but she didn't. She was kind and patient. She knew I was hurting in many ways. She'd put some pads on the mattress, help me to bed, and even put a bowl on my bedside table just in case I needed to throw up. Eventually, we'd both fall asleep hoping that there wouldn't be more messes to clean in the morning, but there often were.

Writing about this after the fact just sounds stupid. Of course, a scenario like this could understandably happen once, or maybe even forgivably twice, but why would I do this to myself multiple times? Why did I so desperately want to get drunk and crazy with my friends like I used to before my accident? Did I need the alcohol as an excuse to be fun or to cry? It was complicated, and it was brutal.

At some point, I knew I had to admit that it just wasn't possible for me to get drunk anymore, and I had to let that go. I had to say goodbye to "party Rob" for my own benefit. And I had to trust that my friends who liked "party Rob" a lot would let him go, too, for my sake. Most importantly, and difficult, would be to remember my own advice in the future should I find myself having consumed three or four beers and wanting to have another. The fourth or fifth drink seemed to be that crucial tipping point when the liquid courage kicked in and all sound reasoning disappeared. At that point, the bender would go into overdrive, and the night would end in a disastrous mess. More accurately, *I'd* end up a disastrous mess.

I knew alcohol was a depressant and that the more I drank, the more likely I was to end up crying on the toilet at the end of the night. So why did I allow myself to open the floodgates to the deepest sadness I'd ever felt? What kind of dysfunctional grieving process was this? What was my problem that I needed to be drunk to cry over what I've lost? I probably should have booked some more sessions with the psychologist.

If alcohol was my gateway drug (easily attainable and socially acceptable to consume with others), I had way too many harder medications available to me as well. Since my accident, I'd been prescribed a plethora of different painkillers, nerve blockers, and antidepressants. I'd typically try a new prescription for a week or two before stopping it because the side effects were worse than any benefits I received. The thing was that I didn't want to throw these medicines in the garbage, so I hung on to them, filling my drawer in the bathroom. Just in case someday I might need something stronger.

Many months and prescriptions later, I had a stockpile of meds that could probably kill a large animal and was being trusted that I wouldn't do anything stupid with them. Rarely did I ever think to take these harder meds. But when I was drunk and depressed, the mere presence of these pills in the house became a potential recipe for tragedy. Of course, I should have just found a way to dispose of these meds. But more importantly, I had to stop being an idiot and drinking my face off.

My girls depended on me, and the drunken notion I had a few times that because I was inebriated that I might be forgiven for hurting myself was unacceptable, childish. I had to do better, so if my friends decided to party on like we used to, it would have to happen without me.

I lost the ability to walk, the ability to control my bowels and bladder. Lost sexual function and the ability to drink away my problems. It was a hell of a shit list that I could trace back to my spinal cord injury. But those were all facts. What I did with them and how I framed them was totally in my control. The accident may have broken my back, but it hadn't broken my spirit. I didn't want to hide away from life. I wanted to get out there, be active, and live the life I'd always imagined.

It was time for me to get back into training.

Chapter 7
Training in All its Forms

"Pain is universal, suffering is optional." – Buddhist saying

I've always looked at the pain that comes from a hard workout or race as "good pain." It's the shot of endorphins that come from pushing my body to its limit, and it's something that I strive for when I work out. It may sound odd or even sadistic, but it's empowering to know that if I'm going to be in pain, then at least it will be the pain of my choosing. To some degree, I'm in control of it, and I know that over time I'll be stronger and faster for my efforts.

I think being the youngest child in my family shaped this perspective towards training and suffering. This combined with my natural inclination to challenge myself to do things that maybe I shouldn't. I remember well the need to do anything my big brothers or sister did, even if it wasn't necessarily age-appropriate. And I believe this drive has been a mostly positive quality throughout my life.

Of course, one could argue that this trait played a role in my poor decision to try that jump in the forest. But that was more a mistake born from haste combined with a lot of bad luck. I believe an accomplishment that is truly great will require hard work and that it will almost always be accompanied by some level of pain.

From the moment I broke my back, I felt like that little child again, needing to do everything my brothers and sisters did no matter who told me I couldn't. The doctors called it rehabilitation but, to me, I was in training. My physical life had started over, and I was determined to learn how to do everything again, but with just the use of my arms. I'd take the pain to make the gains.

Early into my rehab at Lyndhurst, I started pushing myself beyond the expectations others set for me. As mentioned in the previous chapter, a rehab protocol was to have three goals to work towards and getting my driver's license back was my first goal. My second goal was to be fitted for as many sports wheelchairs and handcycles as possible, and I had started that before leaving Lyndhurst. The third and last goal I defined for myself was wanting to learn more wheelchair skills than anyone who had ever left Lyndhurst before.

It didn't take long to realize that the world is full of obstacles for someone trying to get around in a wheelchair. I hated the idea of not being able to go somewhere or do something because of inaccessibility. While at rehab with all these experts and seasoned wheelchair users flying around the place who could show me what's possible, I knew I had to learn everything I could, as quickly as I could, so that when I was out in the bigger world, I'd be able to get over and through any obstacles that I encountered, either by myself or with the help of others.

When I shared this goal with my medical team, much to my surprise, they suggested that I lower my goals or expectations, proposing that instead of writing down "learning the most wheelchair skills" in my file that I settle for "learning a lot of wheelchair skills." I was so disappointed. What the hell? Why would they discourage me like that? Why do I have to be the one challenging them to set the bar high? I'm willing to do the work to achieve the goals I set for myself. Why wouldn't they be on board?

I immediately decided to focus on myself and to humour them. Screw it; it didn't matter. They could write down whatever they wanted. I had my goals, and I was going to accomplish them. They could join me or watch—up to them.

Though it was the third goal I listed, mastering my wheelchair was the first one I could pursue at Lyndhurst. I wheeled around the gym and physiotherapy areas asking the OTs and PTs not assigned to me if they might have a few minutes to give me extra advice and to spot me on wheelchair skills. Skills like taking a fast push at a six-inch curb and trying to get up it or pulling myself backwards up a flight of stairs in my chair. These things took a lot of practice and coaching before they became doable. I wasn't sure if they'd ever become second nature, but I would try.

Every other day or so, I'd set aside time to go down to the gym to work out. Like a treadmill for runners, I spent time on the rollers in my wheelchair, trying to make my pushing muscles stronger. Like a bicycle on the wall, I used the ergometer to get my heart rate up while thinking about one day having my own handcycle. And I tried the different weight machines, working on building strength for all of my many different and frequent transfers. I was working hard, and I was focused.

I went swimming for the first time at the Sunnybrook pool beside Lyndhurst. And it wasn't enough to just be in the water. First time out, I insisted on trying every swimming stroke I knew how to do before my accident. Needless to say, I drank a lot of water that day. And I confirmed that there was no way I was ever going to be able to do a butterfly stroke using just my arms. That stroke was tough enough when I was able-bodied. Sabrina and I had a good laugh watching me try, though.

One day at lunch, a fellow patient who broke his neck falling off a trampoline had heard about my aspirations to become a triathlete before my accident. He enthusiastically assured me that I could still be a triathlete. I'd be a paratriathlete. He went on to tell me about a paratriathlete who lived in Ottawa, named Chris Bourne, and he encouraged me to reach out to him.

Chris was an innovator in the sport and one of the world's best paratriathletes. After lunch, I went to my room, jumped on the internet, found Chris's contact info, grabbed my cell phone, and called him. Much like Rich, Chris was kind and caring and encouraging. He was excited to share with me how one does paratriathlons and how I could get started.

"You can totally do this," Chris told me. "Just let me know how I can help." This phone call started another long and important friendship with an exceptional person. I was so glad someone told me about Chris and that I was confident enough to reach out.

Having left Lyndhurst and getting settled in at home, I wasn't sure if being home was easier or harder for Sabrina. But I knew without a doubt that I was happy to be back with my girls and freed from the confines of a hospital.

At home, the work of figuring out my life really started. The girls were five and three years old now. And while they were learning how to be little responsible and capable persons, it truly felt like I, too, had to learn all the basic physical things in life again, this time from a wheelchair. One of my biggest challenges was relearning how to take care of the girls by myself. Everything physical about being a dad was suddenly much more complicated and difficult. Little things I would never have imagined, like how to give Chloe and Zara a bath. Because I couldn't bend over the bathtub for fear of falling out of my chair into the tub, my solution was to let them have stand-up showers in my roll-in shower instead. This worked great!

Even something as simple as going for a walk around the pond behind our house was interesting. It was one of those February days where the temperature was above freezing, and the snow had started to melt. Chloe was in school, and Zara was keen to get outdoors. Sabrina encouraged me to try out my new all-terrain wheelchair. It was heavier than my normal day chair, with wider mountain bike tires on it that allowed me to go over more surfaces. The plan was for Zara to ride her tricycle, and I'd go for a push.

Once bundled up, we headed down the sidewalk and through the walkway to the pond. The paved parts were no problem. But all of the other surfaces like gravel or crushed stone were wet and spongy, making it incredibly hard for me to push through. It felt like I was in quicksand, or as though all four tires had gone flat at the same time. Little Zara motored over it in her trike. I sank into the muck. There was little rolling and, of course, no coasting. I struggled forward a few inches at a time while little Zara watched with curiosity at my challenge.

Eventually, I made it out of the soft stuff and back onto pavement at the top of the path. It had been a slog, but we did it. And it was fun to be out with my little girl. Me in my wheelchair, her on her tricycle. I was exhausted but happy to be doing dad things again.

A walk around the pond was just the start of relearning how to do my part around the house. I challenged myself to figure out how to pick up Chloe from school, cook a meal, do some woodworking in my shop, and even how to build a snowman with the girls. There was always a memorable story of something going wrong the first time I tried something new. But ultimately, I achieved the goals I set for myself.

And the more I could do for myself at home, the more I was propelled forward in my strength, coordination, confidence, and endurance. This was all training, even if I didn't know it at the time. Getting my life to some semblance of normal was the goal, and the challenges of doing so set me up to pursue the sport-related challenges that awaited me.

A week or two after coming home from Lyndhurst, I learned that Spinal Cord Injury Ontario would be hosting a ski day the following month. The opportunity to get back to a ski hill and try a sit-ski got me excited. I got my doctor's permission to go and planned the outing with Sabrina.

When I first met Rich, the picture he showed me of him flying through the air in his sit-ski had made a big impression on me. He told me that one of the reasons he liked skiing so much was because it allowed him to flirt with gravity and win. He likened it to the feeling of leaning a motorbike through a corner. There was also the element of danger. It required you to temper the thrill of racing downhill with the knowledge that things could go disastrously wrong.

The first couple runs were on the beginner hills. They were fun but not terribly exciting. A few different volunteers tried to explain how to use the sit-ski effectively. The instruction seemed to make sense. But honestly, I was more interested in going to the bigger hills and getting more speed than perfecting my technique on a piece of equipment that was really challenging to master. I didn't have enough time that day to really learn how to sit-ski without someone holding my sit-ski up, so I was fine with just experiencing the thrill.

Just as I had that thought, Scott, one of the volunteers, realized we had a mutual friend, and he asked: "Didn't you used to race motorcycles?" I smiled back at him. "Then I'm taking you to the biggest hills!" he said with enthusiasm. I was game. Fantastic! Let's do this!

Within minutes, and under the supervision and control of Scott and another volunteer, I was flying down the big hills, carving up the slopes and doing high-speed passes next to the cameraman for the money shots. It was amazing. I felt alive. What an excellent day of fun. I was grateful for the opportunity, and I was eager to do more activities like this.

Not long after ski day, Rich delivered to me my very own handcycle. We had ordered it when I was still at Lyndhurst in rehab. I set it up on my stationary trainer from my old mountain bike and started training every day. It felt so good working up a sweat.

With the arrival of spring, I was finally able to take my handcycle off the trainer and outside for a ride. Sabrina and I started with shorter 5 km and 10 km rides around the neighbourhood. I had to remind myself that it wasn't that long ago that I broke my back and that I should pace myself and my expectations. It made sense that I was quick to tire and wouldn't be able to maintain the speeds that I used to with my legs. Regardless though, Sabrina and I were both excited to be outside exercising again, and I loved the feeling of moving again at speed under my own power.

The first week I was home from rehab, even before my handcycle was delivered, I had registered for the second annual Ride to Conquer Cancer. This was a two-day, 200 km charity bicycle ride from Toronto to Niagara Falls. I was excited and nervous about being the first person to attempt this using a handcycle, especially considering I didn't own one yet, and this was a distance I'd never done in my life. Knowing I had five months to figure it out and that I'd be doing the ride with two good friends gave me something momentous to look forward to. Again, having something positive to focus on and train for was good for my health, physically and mentally.

As with all these athletic firsts since my accident, I started slow and short and added speed and distance over time. Living on the West side of Oakville was great because I could venture out of the city and ride up and down the Niagara Escarpment from my home. I'd often done this on my road bike before the accident, but it was different on the handcycle. Climbing hills on a piece of equipment that is at least twice as heavy as a regular bike while using just my arms was incredibly difficult. Sometimes on the steepest hills, I had to stop multiple times to rest and regain my strength before attempting to climb a few more feet. But I never failed to get to the top. I did it as a leap of faith or, perhaps, out of reckless abandon. The important part was that I always found a way.

Riding a handcycle alongside cars and trucks was scary. Lying on my back with my head only 18 inches above the surface of the road, a vehicle is likely to roll right over me rather than push me out of the way. Of course, I had a tall flag and bright LED lights on the front and back, but motorists often buzzed by, leaving only a foot or two of space between their vehicle and me.

Venturing out onto country roads, it didn't take long to get a variety of reactions from motorists. Everything from an encouraging toot of the horn and a thumbs up to expressions of genuine concern from people who asked me to be even more visible. Then there was the time that a farmer on his tractor slowly crept past me on some sleepy backroad, only to turn around and give me the finger. Another time, a plumber in his branded van leaned out his window to yell at me: "Get the fuck off the road!" That exchange made it immediately onto my social media and was followed up with a lot of nasty calls from my friends to the owner of that company, who insisted that his guys would never do that.

One day, I was climbing a hill when a car pulled alongside me. I was on Rattlesnake Road, one of the toughest climbs up the Niagara Escarpment. The young guy driving lowered his window and asked if I had any idea how steep and difficult the road up ahead was. I thanked him and laughed it off. There's no way to know if I can do it or not unless I try, so onward and upward. I may have had to pause a couple of times to make it to the top, but nothing was going to stop me. Cresting that hill was a significant boost to my pride and confidence.

The handcycle is so long that it can't turn very tightly or quickly. It's usually a five- to nine-point-turn to do a 180. So trying to do it on a steep hill means you'd likely get hit by a car coming over the hill. That's assuming that you didn't already tip over sideways and roll all the way down. When you start a hill on a handcycle, you're committed to getting up it. Getting off and walking is never an option.

As hard as it was to climb in the handcycle, I always focused on the fact that what goes up must come down. I still loved speed, and in the first few months, I discovered I could hit over 60 km/h coming down the escarpment. This rush kept me coming back for more.

June came quickly, and with it, the Conquer Cancer ride. It was a beautiful, sunny morning, and I was feeling great. I was a mix of nerves and excitement, but knowing I was riding with my friends put me at ease. They'd take care of me whatever happened.

As I attached my flag, organized my bottles, and checked the air in my tires, other riders smiled and looked on with curiosity. I wondered what they thought seeing me: some guy in a wheelchair, wearing a cycling jersey and putting together this three-wheel contraption.

One guy walked by and snickered, "That looks comfortable." Another said, "Lying down on the job, eh?" I seriously think these people didn't know I couldn't use my legs, even though I was sitting there in a wheelchair!

I reminded myself that I was the first paraplegic to attempt the ride, so I guess it's not surprising if they'd never seen a handcycle before. I certainly hadn't before my accident. Any comment I received would just fuel my resolve. The energy and excitement of the ride were invigorating. Before the organizers started welcoming riders and announcing the millions of dollars raised, Sabrina and I ventured over to the tent for next year's registration. We signed up to do it together.

Day one was tough. We started at a good pace and quickly made our way through Toronto and Mississauga to Oakville. This was my home turf, but I had never ridden through the rolling hills of Oakville after already riding for 50 km. In fact, I'd never handcycled that far before, and the day was only halfway done.

We slowed our pace slightly but soon found ourselves on top of the escarpment in Ancaster. My friends and I loved speed, so of course, we took off down the hill as fast as we could. The hill was over a kilometre long, and it turned to the right as you descended. Within seconds of starting the decline, our speed exceeded 70 km/h, and we flew by a string of other riders.

Just before reaching the bottom of the hill, a large truck pulled out in front of us unexpectedly. I squeezed the brake hard and smelled the pads and rubber burning. It was a little scary almost running into the back of the truck. But once we were safe, it was mostly disappointing that we had to cut short our speed run. After collecting ourselves, we finished day one with a ten-kilometre climb into Hamilton, where we'd stop for the night with a beer at Mohawk College.

Sunday started well, and we quickly set a good pace for the day. The only snag was a flat tire caused by my brake pad wearing through the sidewall of my tire, likely caused by the truck incident the day before. Once my friends quickly fixed the problem, we pushed up the last big hill of the day and enjoyed the last 40 km that brought us into the finish line beside Niagara Falls.

This entire ride was emotionally powerful. Passing so many residents who stood at the end of their driveways with signs that read: *Cancer Survivor Lives Here – Thank You for Riding!* Or seeing a young dad riding a bike with an empty child seat with a note on the back of the seat that read: *In memory of Michael.* I thought about that for a hard second, losing your child. But then I had to focus on something else before the tears building in my eyes started to fall. The emotions of this ride and the accomplishment were so powerful. It was a good reminder for me of how lucky I was to be alive and doing something meaningful and challenging with my friends.

Pulling into the finishing chute, a great cheer rose from the crowd. My eyes immediately found Sabrina, Chloe and Zara, along with my mom, my sister and her husband, and my nephews. All there to cheer us in. It was a powerful moment. This was the biggest athletic accomplishment of my life thus far, and I did it all with my arms. It had been eight months since I broke my back, and here I was. I'd ridden 200 km in two days and became the first paraplegic athlete to complete this epic ride. I felt I was becoming whole again. I was accomplishing things that were significant to me, and I was getting stronger.

I loved this feeling. I wanted more.

If one wants to become a paratriathlete, a handcycle is used for the cycling portion of the race, and a racing wheelchair is used to complete the run. If you've ever seen the Paralympics, you've likely seen a racing chair. The athlete is kneeling in a bucket/seat over the back two wheels, and the long frame of the chair extends a few feet forward, connecting to a single smaller front wheel.

During the summer of 2009, I borrowed a racing chair from Ontario Wheelchair Sports Association. I met a representative at a storage space in Toronto and was invited to find a chair that fit me. I found one that I thought would work and dismantled it to fit into my car.

Once I got home, I was eager to give it a spin. I put air in the tires and pulled on my special wheelchair racing pushing gloves with my teeth that I had purchased online. These gloves were made from thick leather with rubber pads to protect your hands. Sabrina helped me into the chair and handed me my helmet.

It's crazy difficult getting into the racing chair. Folding my long legs in the bucket underneath me, ensuring my feet aren't close to the spokes of the wheels, and keeping everything away from the metal frame so as to avoid skin sores. Unable to feel or move my lower body, all of this needs to happen while I'm transferring my entire body weight from my day chair to the racing chair. It's exhausting.

Thankfully, Sabrina was there to move things around into what we thought was the correct position while also making sure I didn't flip over backwards. The balance point in this chair is in front of the rear axle, which allows a slight amount of weight on the front wheel to steer. However, if you sit up straight in the chair and move your centre of gravity behind the balance point, you're going over backwards in a hurry.

My street had a slight incline, so I was facing uphill for my first ride. With a deep breath and a "here goes nothing" attitude, I pushed on the rubber push rims on the chair with my special padded gloves. It was incredibly tough to apply enough force into the push rim and then push the entire wheel forward, even on the very slight incline of my street. I barely got twenty metres before I questioned what the hell I had gotten myself into. This was the hardest thing I'd done since pushing around the pond with Zara through the soggy ground.

Leaning over with my chest almost parallel to the ground, I strained to hold my head up to see where I was going. Fortunately, I wasn't going that fast and didn't need to worry about running into anyone. My neck muscles were not accustomed to holding my head in that position for very long, and it didn't take long to feel them burning.

After 1.5 km of pushing away from home, I decided to head back. I stopped and rocked the chair back and forth multiple times, trying to pop the front wheel off the ground just enough to coax the chair into doing a 180-degree turn. Having managed that, I anticipated the rush of speed that was to come.

Even though it was just a gentle slope, I immediately started gaining speed. I also quickly realized that the racing chair worked differently than the handcycle. As the rear wheels turned faster, my pushes to maintain control lost their effectiveness. I had to rely on the spring-loaded front wheel steering and single brake to avoid hitting anything or anyone. It wasn't easy.

Trying to steer away from parked cars and the curb, I tried thrusting my gloves down on the rims as hard and as fast as I could. Doing so, I immediately learned a painful lesson about this chair. When you forcefully thrust your hands down to the pushing rims and miss, it's likely that the soft tissue on the inside of your arms will touch the quickly turning rubber push rim. When this happens, that sensitive skin is quickly removed. It's like a burn from an iron. It hurts like hell.

At this moment, though, I was too excited and encouraged by the speed to worry about a little skin burn. I quickly found myself in front of my house and engaged the front brake—the only brake on this particular wheelchair. I then learned my third lesson of the day. It turns out that the brakes on a racing chair are more for show than anything else. They should be called "slight speed modulators" because that's really all they can do.

Pulling the brake lever tight with the inside of my gloves stopped the front wheel from turning, but it didn't stop the chair from moving. I skidded past my house and then a couple of my neighbours' houses before finally coming to a stop.

These were all things I would have to keep in mind going forward, and they were all things I learned on my first "racing wheelchair" run. On the shitty side, it was really tough, it was painful, and you had very little control. But this chair allowed you to join in running races, and it could be fast and exciting. I'd focus on the positives.

During that summer, I hooked up with a local wheelchair racing team. They were called the McWheelers and coached by Ken Thom. His son Curtis, a Paralympian, and a few other young racers, all welcomed me into the group and gave me advice and pointers that they thought I might find helpful. I was certainly the old guy in the group but was happy to be included and learning this sport from experienced athletes.

When October arrived, Sabrina and I drove to Ottawa to race in the Colours Half-Marathon. This was our second half-marathon ever and the first for me in the racing wheelchair.

The morning was crisp and cold, but we knew we'd soon warm up once we started moving. We gave each other a kiss and wished each other luck as the announcer counted down from ten to start the race. We were off.

The first kilometre of the race was downhill. This should have been fast and fun, but it turned out to be difficult and frustrating. Instead of flying down the hill leading the runners, I found myself behind a mass of runners trying everything at my disposal to prevent myself from running into them from behind. My front wheel brake didn't work well enough, so I grabbed both of my rear wheels to slow myself down. Even with my thick leather gloves on, it wasn't long before I had to modulate my grip to prevent my hands from burning from all the friction. This was not a good start.

I tried yelling, "Wheelchair on the left!" hoping that runners would move out of the way. But they either failed to hear me or just didn't care. I was fortunate not to hit anyone.

At the bottom of the first hill, I turned right to see a long and steep string of hills ahead. It was almost 8 km of climbing and over 60 metres (200 feet) of elevation! My god.

I quickly confirmed there were few things more difficult than climbing hills in a racing chair, especially for a newbie. Think about riding a single-speed bicycle up a steep hill. Now imagine pedalling that bike with your arms. There's no mechanical assistance; you just have to gut it out.

I let my head hang down as I didn't dare look at the entire hill; that was too daunting. Instead, I grabbed the outside of my wheels and cranked away, ten inches at a time. Many runners asked if I wanted a push, which was kind. But I couldn't accept. This was something I had to do on my own. After what felt like an hour, I crested the hill.

The next 8 km were a series of mostly rollers that allowed me to pick up the pace. That was followed by a long and fast downhill to the finish. I finished my first half-marathon in a time of 1:45:10. That was nine minutes faster than my first half-marathon just before my accident!

My neck was seized from trying to hold my head up to see where I was going for so long, and the skin on my hands was raw where it had blistered and torn away, but I had done it. I could compete in and complete running races again. I just had to use my chair and suck up a lot of pain.

As 2009 came to an end, I had accomplished several goals that I had set for myself. This included going back to work part time at Microsoft after being away for eight months. My professional life was such a big part of my identity before my accident that getting back to work and picking up where I left off was important to me.

As I expected, everyone at the office was welcoming and accommodating. They seemed happy to have me back. And when they knew for certain that I didn't want any special consideration because of my injury, they were quick to pile on the work. I invited it and urged my manager to keep giving me more, despite her reservations. I had to prove to myself that I could do it all, regardless of how much harder it was to maintain the quality and volume of work I used to complete while still learning to live with a spinal cord injury.

Officially I was allowed to work 20 hours a week. By the end of 2010, I was much closer to 40. My dream of moving to Redmond to work for Microsoft was still alive, but it was incredibly daunting and complicated. Here at home, I had so many family members and friends helping to make my world accessible. Moving abroad would be a whole other complex endeavour. I'd shelve that plan for a little while but feel good knowing that it still could potentially happen someday.

It wasn't just Microsoft that took a lot of my time. Early that year, I also wanted to learn how to swim long distances again. My good friend Peter was a member of Milton's Masters' Swim Team, and he invited me to attend the open swim hour before their weekly practice, where he'd try to help me.

The first stroke I wanted to figure out was front crawl. This was how the fastest triathletes swam. Initially, I thought it would have been easy to do. I just wouldn't use my legs to kick. What I quickly learned was that when I tried to swim forward using just my arms, my legs sank like an anchor towards the bottom of the pool because I have no abdominals to keep my body straight in the water. This prevented me from moving forward at all.

The first day we played with some floatation devices that were around the pool area. But for the second trip to the pool, I brought Chloe's small lifejacket with me. Holding the jacket upside down, Peter helped me thread my legs through the armholes and hiked it up as high as we could. With this added buoyancy, my lower body was closer to the surface of the water, allowing me to move forward slowly. It took a few swim sessions to make any progress, but eventually, I started figuring out my version of the front crawl. To breathe, I swept my hand to the inside of my body at the end of my pull, which helped to turn my torso on my side just long enough so that when I turned my head too, I could sneak a breath and carry on. It wasn't pretty, but I was swimming.

Another challenge I had with swimming resulted from the two titanium rods in my back. These rods have a bend in them, similar to someone slouching at their desk. As a result, my spine holds the shape of a turtle's shell. The consequence of this is that when I'm on my front in the water, my face is pushed under the surface. This makes sighting and turning to breathe extra difficult.

It took several trips to the pool to experiment and figure out how to overcome these challenges. With a lot of help from Peter, a custom pair of wetsuit pants for even more buoyancy, and a ton of persistence, I was eventually able to swim 2 km of laps nonstop by the spring of 2010.

As August approached, I knew I could swim without drowning, handcycle 100 km in a day, and push a hilly half-marathon. I had all the skills and equipment needed to attempt my first triathlon. I just needed to put them all together on the same day.

I reached out to the organizers of the Wasaga Olympic Triathlon scheduled for the beginning of September. John, the owner of Multisport Canada Triathlon, was thrilled that I wanted to compete in his race and worked with his team and me to make sure all three disciplines and transitions of the race were accessible. To make the day even more exciting, Peter signed up with me. He was an accomplished and powerful swimmer and cyclist, but he wasn't a runner. This was going to be interesting for both of us.

The second weekend of September came quickly. Awake at 4:00 AM, I got dressed, ate breakfast, and headed out of the house as quietly as I could. I picked up Peter in Georgetown, and we were on our way. Wasaga Beach is a picturesque little town on the eastern edge of Lake Huron. As we drove north, the sun slowly rose to reveal one of those warm, sunny weekends that feel like an extension of summer.

Every race morning brings with it the usual pre-competition jitters and nerves. I think that's part of why we sign up for these things. It's that excitement, combined with the finisher's medal waiting for you, that drives you to compete. This race morning was more intense than any other race I had experienced before. My jitters were multiplied times three. My mind was consumed with trying to confirm that I had my equipment, logistics, and strategy to swim, bike and run in the same race, all sorted out.

Twenty minutes before the start, Peter and another racer helped me into my wetsuit and down to the edge of the lake. It must have rained the night before because the beach sand was flat, damp, and compacted. That made it easier to roll on, and I could get right down to the water's edge in my wheelchair.

The water was shallow for about 50 metres before it got deeper where the racecourse started. Despite the sunny weather, the cool water had a bite to it. Fortunately, the wetsuit kept me comfortable, and I knew that soon I'd be working hard. As I bobbed there in the water with my head just above the surface, the buoys that marked our destination suddenly seemed really far away. Oh shit.

We were doing an Olympic distance triathlon. That's a 1.5 km swim followed by a 40 km bike ride and finishing with a 10 km run. There are shorter distance triathlons, but I figured that if I was going to do this, I wanted each discipline to be a challenge.

The horn sounded for our wave to start. I didn't want to get in people's way, so I let the other swimmers get ahead of me. I was happy to be doing the triathlon, but I knew I wouldn't be able to keep up during this portion of the competition. My swimming and sighting skills left a lot to be desired, and I hadn't really received any formal coaching at this point.

My goal for the swim was to stay focused and go as fast as I could without burning out (or drowning). When I got tired, I could do a backstroke to catch my breath. The short rest was helpful, but being on my back was problematic as it allowed the Cliff bar and Gatorade I'd had on shore to regurgitate into my mouth. This, of course, forced me to turn back onto my stomach, spit, and carry on with the front crawl.

After the second or third time this happened, I reflected on how I was glad there wasn't anyone behind me that would have to swim through my throw-up. Around that same time, I remembered that I was one of the slowest swimmers out there and that many triathletes pee in the water before finishing their swim. So, maybe I was the one that should be worried.

Peter did the swim at a time of 27:36. He ran over the swim-exit timing mat to record his swim time and then waited for me. While searching for me in the distance, he recruited a spectator to help bring me from the sandbar to my wheelchair. They positioned the chair at the edge of the water, and once I was sitting and balanced, Peter hauled me backwards through the swim finish chute. The sand that had been hard-packed before the race had been churned up by all the swimmers running out of the water, and it was now more like quicksand. Peter was in amazing shape, but he had to haul me through wet sand, still wearing his wetsuit, in the midst of doing a whole triathlon. Spectators cheered us on, and I went across the swim timing mat at 44:48.

I had fallen behind most of the other competitors in the swim, but I got back into my groove on the handcycle. I rode strategically, trying to keep my heart rate in the low 160s. The Wasaga bike course was mostly flat, with the exception of one reasonably sized hill. I felt my heart rate increase for the hill climb, but I was able to bring it under control for the rest of the ride. I did the 40 km in 1:34:03, averaging 25.5 km/h. That was my best average speed to date.

There was no one in transition when I arrived. Just a sea of bikes as all the athletes were already on the run portion of the race. I had to get from my handcycle into my wheelchair and then from my wheelchair into my racing chair. I looked around for someone to potentially help me and got lucky.

The run course started off on the narrow boardwalk along the beach and then went onto the residential side streets of Wasaga. At the end of the boardwalk, runners stepped over a curb and ran on a short section of grass trail to cut the corner of the course. In my racing chair, this wasn't an option, so I stayed on the streets and took the long way around.

The running course consisted of two 5 km loops, so once I got on the course, there were runners all around me, many on their second lap. Between the runners and the cars on the sections of the road that were not closed, I found myself battling traffic the entire run. Upon seeing me in my racing chair pushing as hard as I could, drivers didn't know whether to stop and let me pass or to race past me. A mix of the two happened.

Avoiding cars, runners and curbs definitely added some extra stress and navigational work, but it didn't matter. I was just so elated to have the end of my first triathlon in sight that I didn't care if I was dodging oncoming traffic or pedestrians making their lazy way to a day on the beach. I even started passing many of the athletes I had been chasing all swim and bike—including Peter—which was so awesome! I was flying in my racing chair.

I finished my 10+ km run in 35:20, completing my first-ever triathlon in a total time of 3:08:10. What a feeling! Peter came in shortly after me, and we celebrated by chugging one-litre cartons of chocolate milk that he had brought from home. It was the perfect day, and I was hooked!

The thrill of going fast and pushing my limits went beyond the triathlon. My "need for speed" was alive and well, and I desperately wanted to get back onto the racetrack, my happy place. Before my accident, motorcycling was by far my greatest passion. The thrill of riding around a track at over 250 km/h and dragging my knee in the corner hit all my senses hard. My new car, the Infiniti G37s, was quick, and until I could figure out how to ride a motorcycle again, it would have to do. At my first opportunity, I signed up for a track day at Mosport, just over an hour away from home.

At the track, the drivers were sorted into three groups: beginner, intermediate and advanced. I self-selected intermediate, as I knew the racetrack well and was confident that I'd be able to keep up. While I had done countless laps over the last 15 years on the motorbikes, driving the track in my car was a new experience. I asked for an instructor to come with me and give me advice, which many different instructors were happy to do. As it turned out, the car was much easier to get around the track than the motorcycles. The car was quick, but it didn't accelerate or brake anywhere nearly as quickly as any of the motorbikes I'd owned. Add to that the comfort and confidence of being strapped to the driver's seat inside what's essentially a cage with airbags, and the concerns and worry of hurting yourself almost disappeared.

My first few laps were comfortable and easy, by track day standards. I reminded myself repeatedly not to rush things. I had all day to find the limits of me and my car, but only if I wasn't reckless. Learning the braking and turn-in points to carry the maximum amount of speed at the apex was key to a good lap. And as my pace rapidly improved, I discovered that I had two important issues to solve. The first was keeping my torso in the driver's seat, and the second was ensuring I didn't lose my brakes going into corners.

Driving on the street, the throttle and brake are controlled with my left hand, and I steer and balance myself with my right. Driving on the racetrack with speed and forces magnified, new variables are introduced into the equation. Turning hard to the right was still fine, as I could brace my body on the driver's door with my left shoulder and arm. But braking hard, turning to the left, and especially turning to the left while braking hard, things got dicey.

On the street, I could hold my upper body secure mid-left-turn by ensuring my right hand was between 12 and 3 o'clock on the steering wheel at the apex. At the track, though, when travelling at speed and braking or turning hard, the G-forces were amplified, and my entire body was pulled towards the passenger seat. As strong as my arms were, I was unable to steer accurately and hold myself securely at the same time. To keep from losing my balance and crashing, I needed a second strap to hold me in my driver's seat.

Thinking that could be an issue for me, I had thrown an old suitcase luggage strap from home into the car before heading out to the track. Fastening this strap around my chest and the back of the seat and cinching it tight, I then felt safe and secure, planted in my seat and now able to use my arms and hands for just controlling the car. I amused myself, having just come up with what was essentially a do-it-yourself five-point harness.

The second issue I had to solve came as a big surprise when I tried to apply the brakes at the end of the straight, and they only partially worked. What the hell?! I quickly glanced down and saw that my left foot had slid under the brake pedal, and as I pushed the brake pedal down with my hand control, I was squishing my shoe and my foot between the pedal and the floor. Replacing my right hand with my left on the steering wheel, I used my right hand to quickly dislodge my foot so I could get full braking before going off the corner. A scary moment, but exactly the kind of adrenaline-producing experience I expected from a track day. I pulled into the pits to solve this before carrying on.

Reaching into the back seat, I grabbed a couple of beach towels that I kept in the car to dry my wheels on wet days. Strategically wrapping the towels under, around, and between my legs, I hoped that doing this would prevent my legs and feet from sliding around anymore in the turns. It wasn't perfect, but it worked.

By the end of the day, I had rediscovered my track day groove and enjoyed the thrill of finding my limits and those of my car. And in the process, I passed a wide variety of nicer cars, including Porsches, Audis, BMWs, and even a few exotics that were faster cars on paper but being driven by more tentative guys. It was a great day.

Leaving the track, I turned onto the secondary highway towards home and started crying. Surprised at myself, I questioned why. Why that after such a great day of racing around the track was my next emotion tears? I guessed in some way they were tears of joy. I hadn't realized how much I missed the thrill of going fast. The speed, the sounds, the smells, the fear, the satisfaction of balancing the car and hitting a turn perfectly, the banter with the other guys driving... All of that was such a big part of my life before I broke my back, and even though this day had been on four wheels, the result was the same as two. I still loved going fast, simple as that. I had to do more of this, and in the coming years, I would.

By the end of 2010, I had accomplished so much! I worked hard, I embraced the pain of training and rehab, and I was stronger for it. Home life was good, I was back at work part time, and I could even call myself a paratriathlete. I was approaching that feeling of happiness that I had in 2008, before my accident. It was the feeling that everything seemed too good to be true, and perhaps it was. The height of my successes would soon start to fade away as I was forced to finally face my biggest challenge.

Chapter 8

The Cruelest Pain

It first happened in rehab. I noticed a tingling feeling in my feet. I told the doctors about it, hopeful that this could be the start of recovering sensation in my lower body. But they weren't so optimistic. They told me I was most likely experiencing neuropathic pain, and they wrote me a prescription for some medication that was supposed to make it manageable.

I looked up the diagnosis online, and the first thing I learned is that neuropathic pain is also known as suicide pain. Not a great start. My search yielded articles that were disjointed, inaccessible, and vague. It quickly became clear that no one had a reliable solution to this problem.

Neuropathic pain is caused by damage to the nervous system, resulting in moderate to intense chronic pain. The modalities most often promoted to help reduce this pain are pharmaceutical, like antidepressants in low dosages. For some people, these have been shown to ease neuropathic pain as a side effect of treating some other ailment or condition, but I'd learn that for me, they created more problems than they solved. Medications for neuropathic pain typically impact your overall mental well-being, and to date, their efficacy rates for treating it are very low. When no known cure or remedy exists, doctors are resigned for you to try anything and everything.

I've always tried to be a positive person. But when you learn that loss of mobility is probably not the worst result of a spinal cord injury—and that there is little knowledge and fewer existing solutions to help you with a pain so intense it is known to cause suicides—it makes you wonder why solving this problem isn't more of a priority.

The doctors started me on a drug called Gabapentin, an anti-seizure drug that might numb nerve pain when taken in small dosages. But they prefaced this recommendation with a warning that I would probably have to try a lot of different medications, dosages, and combinations before I found something that actually provided some relief.

On a typical day during the first few years, I'd wake up in the morning pain-free. Maybe there was a tingling in my lower body, but nothing to complain about. Unfortunately, as the day wore on, the tingling would turn into a burning sensation that would get progressively worse with each hour. Over the course of the day, the intensity of the burning increased until my entire lower body, from my chest down, felt like it was on fire. There were nights I couldn't sleep at all because of the pain. If I was lucky enough to catch a few minutes of rest, I'd wake in the morning already in excruciating pain.

People have different experiences of neuropathic pain. For me, it feels like my skin is on fire from my chest down. There's no explanation for it. I can touch my leg with my hand and feel that the skin is not burning; it may even be cold if I've been outside or in the basement. But the pain signals generated in my brain are telling my consciousness there's a serious problem happening that needs to be dealt with immediately. My body is ready to fight or flee. These signals are incredibly convincing, and there's nothing I can do to calm them. My only hope is to get through the day, have a good night's sleep, and hopefully, when I wake the next day, the pain will be reset and gone.

My primary goal when I left rehab was to get my life back to normal. Or as normal as possible, considering my new challenges. Solving the neuropathic pain was just one of the items on my to-do list. At first, I trusted that managing this pain would be like building endurance for a sporting event. With enough time and persistence, I'd generate a tolerance to the pain so that it wouldn't bother me.

Being back to work part time while trying to add as many hours and responsibilities as quickly as my manager would let me started to take its toll towards the end of 2010. Being away from the office while recovering at home, I realized how much I missed the people, the pace, and the challenges that come with Microsoft. The work environment had been tough but rewarding when I was able-bodied. And I was sure that if I could replicate my ability to add value—but do it from a wheelchair—I'd be unstoppable.

I loved being back in the office with my peers. But unfortunately, I wasn't able to outwork the neuropathic pain. With every passing week, it slowly increased. In those moments at work when I had the opportunity to pause and take a breath, the pain was just waiting for me to admit its presence. If I acknowledged that I experienced the burning, I'd have the immediate sensation of being dropped into a tub of boiling water.

In some ways, the fast pace of Microsoft offered escape. Consumed with solving work-related problems and tasks left me very little time to contemplate how my body felt. There was just too much work to do and opportunities to seize to allow your brain to wander.

Without a doubt, my accident sent me chasing after the stress of deadlines to distract myself from my pain. I've always imposed certain expectations on myself that propelled me throughout my academic and work careers. That jolt of adrenaline that powers all-nighters—that allows you to achieve amazing things—is addictive. But there was another brutal surprise awaiting me.

After my injury, this stress that had once fueled my ability to work under pressure now fueled my neuropathic pain. The greater the stress, the more I felt like I was on fire. It didn't make sense. I was trying to get my life back to normal, and I was physically doing everything I needed to with just my arms. But this nerve pain—this fake pain in my head—had become my biggest nemesis. It was a cruel joke. The part of my body that I couldn't feel or move was the part of my body that seemed to hurt me the most. Even when, rationally, I could see that, physically, my body looked fine.

I worked at Microsoft as much as I could until the end of 2010, at which time I had to concede that my pain wasn't getting any better and my overall health was deteriorating. I made the decision to go on Long-Term Disability so that I could focus all my energy on solving my nerve pain once and for all. If I could do that, the world would once again offer possibilities.

Having completed 18 months back at Microsoft, I felt that I had proven to myself that I could do my job. But I also had to admit that work was the only thing I could do if I kept working. The more I worked, the less time I spent with my girls, my friends, or my sports. Living with a disability meant that everything took more time, which just made everything harder. For my whole life, I'd defined my identity through being a productive, hardworking professional. But now, I needed to prioritize my health and quality of life over this other part of my identity. I said goodbye to my colleagues on the last day before the Christmas holidays in 2010 and haven't been back to work since.

As 2011 started, I had to give myself a new full-time job: solving my neuropathic pain. I had studied statistics in university and grad school, and I did the Six Sigma Black Belt certification during my first consulting job after school. I figured that I should be able to complete some simple correlation calculations over time to see if anything I was doing was effective at reducing my pain.

In simple terms, I created a table and noted my level of nerve pain on a scale of one to ten, three times a day, along with any other time or variable that I thought might impact my pain. My goal was to see, statistically, if anything I did or avoided might have a measurable correlation to the amount of pain I experienced. If I could increase my chances of having a better day with less pain, then that would be progress.

For eight months, I kept a detailed Excel file of my pain levels and everything I did each day. Variables that I thought might impact my pain included the amount of time I slept at night and napped during the day, how long I exercised versus how long I spent on the computer, any therapies or treatments I had, how much caffeine or alcohol I drank, and, of course, the different medications I was prescribed and their dosages.

Early on, I tried meditation and Reiki, but they just made me fall asleep. I visited the chiropractor and a massage therapist. And while that helped tremendously with the physical pain I had from my injury and the increasing amounts of triathlon training I was doing, it often made the neuropathic pain worse.

In 2012, a good friend recommended an acupuncturist in Toronto. He referred to her as "hardcore" and my best chance of getting relief. I made the drive into Toronto, and even though the clinic was difficult to get into in the wheelchair, I made the effort to have seven or eight treatments. For all the effort, the result was more pain. Acupuncture ended badly when I sat up from the table after treatment and couldn't take a deep breath. Each time I tried, pain radiated from my chest all the way through to my back.

I remember hearing once that it was possible for acupuncturists to puncture a lung if they weren't careful, but I really didn't think it would ever happen to me. Especially considering that I'd already had a punctured lung from my accident. I mean, really, who experiences something like that twice in their lifetime?

On the way home, the pain in my chest started to build. I took a Tylenol 3 and rested when I got home. I hoped the pain would subside, that maybe she only hit a nerve or muscle that was extra sensitive. But no luck. After dinner, I called my chiropractor and asked her what she thought. She confirmed the likely diagnosis and recommended I go to the ER immediately.

I arrived at Oakville Hospital ER just after 7:30 PM and told them what I thought the problem was. Either because they didn't hear me or just didn't listen, I spent the next three hours waiting around and having my heart tested. Around 10:30, they told me my heart was fine. I reiterated that it wasn't my heart that was the concern, it was my lungs. Finally, they took a chest x-ray.

After waiting until 1:00 AM, I asked if I could go home. I desperately needed to get out of my wheelchair, use the bathroom, and go to sleep. And on top of everything else, my neuropathic pain was at a ten out of ten. It always seemed to amplify when I was within the walls of a hospital. The ER doctor glanced over my x-ray and said it was fine for me to go home.

When I awoke the next morning, I still had some discomfort in my chest. But I had a 10:00 AM appointment for a hypnosis treatment. I'd never really been interested in alternative medicine before my accident, but I was open to any solution that would help with this pain. Hypnosis seemed like something worth trying based on the logic that my brain might be the gatekeeper of my nerve pain. I knew of smokers who had success quitting after a few hypnosis sessions, and I liked the idea of turning off the pain centres in my brain. In the back of my mind, I wondered if I could use this tactic to improve my performance in sports. Turn off the pain and go faster sounded like a winning plan.

Despite the discomfort in my chest, I decided to carry on with my day as planned. After all, the ER doctor had assured me that everything was fine. In the hypnotist's apartment, I reclined in her chair and settled into a calm and relaxed state. She started her therapy when suddenly there was a loud banging at the apartment door. This was immediately followed by a deep voice asking, "Is Robert Buren in there? This is the Oakville Police!"

The woman raced to the door and opened it. An officer told her that there was an ambulance waiting for Robert downstairs to take him to the hospital.

The hypnotist looked puzzled and asked why I didn't tell her I had been at the hospital the night before. I told her I had an incident that proved to be nothing, so I didn't think it was important to share. The ER doctor said I was fine and sent me home. As I transferred into my chair and headed towards the elevator with my police escort, I heard her mumble under her breath, "I hope this isn't bad for my business." Funny.

Back at the hospital, I learned that the radiologist had come in that morning and reviewed all of the x-rays that had been taken during the night. It was this specialist that confirmed what I feared. The acupuncturist had indeed punctured my lung with a needle, and it was starting to collapse. Fuck! Not again! And not this week!

The doctor gave me two options. Stay and have a chest tube inserted or take it easy at home and come back every week for a follow-up x-ray with the expectation that in four to six weeks, the lung would have healed on its own. After my first experience with a chest tube, there was no question that I'd prefer to let things heal on their own.

Normally, taking a short break from my training and riding would be an okay thing to do. I tend to overdo things, so a forced recovery period might be good. Unfortunately, though, once again, the timing for something like this to happen was terrible. The coming weekend I was to co-lead a team in my third Conquer Cancer Ride from Toronto to Niagara Falls. Our team had raised over a quarter of a million dollars. The riders were a large group of friends, family, and colleagues. It even included Karen, the anesthesiologist that saved me when I was in Hamilton General after my accident, and Keenan, my 14-year-old nephew who bought a road bike and trained just for this event. What a mess. What a disappointment. I'd have to sit on the side of the road and watch. This was torture for me.

Trying hard not to let my disappointment wreck it for anyone else, I worked hard to gain perspective on what this ride was about. It certainly was not about me. Yes, I had my challenges, but this was about all those having fought or currently fighting cancer. I had to be grateful for what I still could do to make this a successful and memorable weekend for everyone, so I decided I'd support the team by taking photos and being there in person at the beginning of the ride, the end of day one, and at the finish line. I was heartbroken to not be able to complete this epic ride again, but I was proud of Sabrina, Keenan and all my teammates for crushing the 200 km in two days. An epic ride indeed.

When friends heard about my punctured lung, they encouraged me to sue the acupuncturist for malpractice. Looking back to the appointments, I realized they were always a little frenetic. She moved very quickly, with what I thought was the confidence of expertise and experience. She bounced around like a pinball from one room to the next, working on as many people as possible in the shortest amount of time.

While some might find this a cause for concern, I really don't think that this itself was the problem. I think things went south when she continued to insert needles into my back while answering the office phone and scheduling appointments to memory. Apparently, she had trouble keeping a receptionist. So rather than let calls go to voicemail, she answered every call herself, holding her phone between her shoulder and head while simultaneously sticking long needles into patients' bodies.

After I called and told her what she'd done, she was surprised and, of course, apologetic. She encouraged me to come for free acupuncture and massage. But going back to that clinic was the last thing I would ever do.

When I considered legal action, I thought back to my first appointment with her. After sharing the challenges that I had with my neuropathic pain, she told me that she didn't have experience treating this kind of pain. But she promised she would try everything she could to help. And if my health insurance did not cover her treatments, she'd treat me for free. She just wanted me to feel better.

Remembering her kind offer, I felt compelled to forgive her for her carelessness. I didn't pursue any kind of compensation from her. In our last conversation, I told her it was unacceptable to be answering the phone while sticking people with needles and that in the future, she'd have to get a receptionist or let the calls go to voicemail. I don't know if she ever did, nor does my good friend (who also never went back). But I hope that she learned something and that the care she provides has improved.

Even still, I needed to find something—anything—that could help me. While none of the non-pharmaceutical options and treatments I'd tried seemed to be helping me, I turned my focus once again to trying to find a pharmaceutical fix.

I went back to my doctors and started with the most commonly prescribed medications to help decrease neuropathic pain. I felt because I had lived with my injury for a couple of years now, perhaps the medications would have a different effect on me. Once again, I played with different prescriptions, combinations and dosages, but like before, nothing provided relief, and the side effects seemed even worse this time around.

As for the physical pain that I could feel within my upper body, this could be managed with medications like Tylenol 3, Arthrotec, or Celebrex. While too much might cause some light-headedness and codeine tends to constipate you, I had no problem taking a pill that provided relief without significant, negative side effects.

Neuropathic pain, however, is much different. I'm not sure anyone knows for certain what causes it. It could be the nerves in the body from below the injury sending actual pain signals up to the brain. Or potentially a misfiring of nerves at the area where the spinal cord is damaged. Perhaps it's just a warning signal generated by the brain, firing pain signals to warn the person that a problem (like not moving my legs) needs fixing ASAP.

In my case, I believed that my brain was freaking out that I hadn't tried to move my lower body since my accident, and it was concerned. To get my attention, it sent the fight or flight adrenaline to my consciousness combined with the sensation of burning pain in the hope that I would change my behaviour and start using those lower-body brain maps again.

Over the years, I learned that chronic pain gets worse over time. Because when the source of the pain is not dealt with, the brain is allowed to use more and more of its processing power—even borrowing from different function centres of the brain—to increase the efficiency and intensity of the pain signals. Your brain becomes an expert at giving you these signals, even though it's totally counterproductive.

The first class of medications that doctors prescribe to try and reduce neuropathic pain was actually developed to ease depression. As it turns out, they found that taking antidepressants like Gabapentin and Nortriptyline in dosages less than those prescribed to treat depression had the effect of easing the neuropathic pain for some patients. It was an opportunistic side effect that might provide relief.

I tried these medications at increasing dosages and combinations, but I didn't get any relief. I then moved on to a newer drug called Pregabalin, which is marketed under the brand name Lyrica. This is one of the newer medications developed for those suffering from ailments such as epilepsy, neuropathic pain, restless leg syndrome, fibromyalgia, and generalized anxiety disorder.

Like any medication I was prescribed, I started Lyrica at the lowest recommended dosage. If I didn't get any relief from the neuropathic pain, I gradually increased the dosage. Before I reached the maximum recommended dosage for Lyrica, I both continued to have neuropathic pain and experienced a number of known side effects. The list of side effects for this drug is long, including (but certainly not limited to) blurred vision, constipation, dizziness, drowsiness, fatigue, headache, and weight gain. In many ways, to risk or even experience these side effects would have been worth it if they helped to lessen my neuropathic pain. But the bigger problem for me was the other side effects.

While on this medicine, I often found myself driving around in my car, evaluating different ways that I could kill myself while making it look like an accident. Maybe I could make driving off a bridge or into a huge tree look like a highspeed mistake of carelessness (everyone knew I loved speed). I was thinking of taking my life, but I couldn't help thinking about how that action would impact the loved ones I'd leave behind. If I did something, I had to be smart about it. Even though I couldn't imagine continuing to live with so much pain, I knew I could never put the pain and burden of suicide on my children. If I took my life, it would have to look like an accident so my children would never know the truth. Their well-being would always be more important than mine.

This thinking scared the hell out of me. I really didn't know why I was having these thoughts or why it felt like they were going to overwhelm me.

As it turns out, there are other reported side effects of Lyrica: cognitive dysfunction, confusion, accidental injury, and neuropathy. Some of the very conditions it was supposed to treat. In my opinion, the label should read: *This probably won't work and might make your symptoms worse. If you don't kill yourself first.*

After eight months of measuring and recording my pain three times a day, I had quantifiable evidence of my suffering. I didn't feel better, nor could I see any statistically meaningful correlations to my pain in the health chart I was keeping, and in fact, the process of recording and thinking about my pain constantly probably made it worse. There's a concept in pain management called catastrophizing, which refers to the way that constant negative thinking about pain exacerbates the experience of it. There's a growing body of research on this subject, and some studies have found that catastrophizing plays a significant role in determining whether pain becomes chronic or not.

I had arrived at an entirely new low. The alternative treatments I tried didn't do anything, and now I was taking medications that allowed my brain to contemplate suicide. It was the darkest time of my life.

Looking for some light to lift me from the darkness, I decided I had to go back to setting goals and accomplishing them. Even if I couldn't get rid of the pain, I could at least distract myself from it and be productive. Of all the things I tried to help me with the pain, exercise was probably the most helpful. When I exercised, I felt and looked better. I ate and slept better. Overall, I was a happier, better person.

As the three-year anniversary of my accident approached, I decided that I would stop taking all my medications and set a fitness-related goal instead. I reminded myself that life and my disability could have been much worse. I could have lost the use of my arms. I could have died. But I didn't. I was still alive and, although I had challenges, I wanted to live. Really live. And do things that were meaningful and significant to me.

I remembered the feeling of completing my first half-marathon before my accident. I wanted that again, but I wanted even more. So, what was it going to be? What athletic goal was significant enough to top what I'd already done? What could distract me from my near-constant neuropathic pain? What was the most difficult physical achievement that I could think of?

There was only one thing that fit the bill.

The Ironman.

Chapter 9

The Road to Kona

I still remember the afternoon, months after my accident. I was lying on my bed flipping through TV channels and came upon a recap of the 2008 Ironman World Championships in Kona, Hawaii. Sabrina and the girls joined me to watch this epic 226 km race in some of the toughest conditions in the world. The heat, the humidity, the wind, and the elevation drew the world's best competitors. I couldn't imagine how hard that must be.

The Ironman World Championship started in 1978, combining the three toughest endurance races in Hawaii. In its inaugural year, fifteen athletes showed up to take the Ironman challenge. According to legend, they were given three sheets containing rules and a course description. But all it said on the last page was: *Swim 2.4 miles! Bike 112 miles! Run 26.2 miles! Brag for the rest of your life!* All that, with a seventeen-hour time limit. Athletes completing an Ironman will burn between 7,000 and 10,000 calories during the race and, in some years, up to a quarter of the athletes will visit the medical tent sometime during the day.

The race takes place on the Big Island of Hawaii, along the Kona coast known for its barren lava fields, *ho'omumuku* crosswinds as strong as 70 km/h, and scorching 35-degree average temperatures. These days, more than two thousand athletes attempt this race each year. It's the ultimate test of body, mind, and spirit, and those who complete it earn the title of Ironman.

In the 2008 Ironman, one of the athletes that NBC followed was a young guy in his twenties from California. His name was Ricky James. Ricky was a motocrosser who broke his back racing a few years earlier, and this was his first Ironman competition. Seeing this handsome young kid swim, handcycle, and push his racing wheelchair to the finish line planted the seed in my mind. The pain, the struggle, the determination, the accomplishment... It made for some very compelling television. But seeing some young Cali kid do it was one thing. Could an older guy like me, recently injured, ever do the same?

I'd never heard of a Canadian paraplegic doing an Ironman race before. But as I was new to the paraplegic community, this wasn't a surprise. I knew of some Paralympic athletes, but they were all focused on the racing chair. I did some online searches and even wrote to the Ironman organization asking them if a Canadian para had ever done a full Ironman. They responded that they didn't keep track of those kinds of stats but to their knowledge, no.

I thought if I could do an Ironman, I could do anything. And if I could be the first Canadian paraplegic to complete the Ironman World Championships in Hawaii, that would be something that would be uniquely mine forever. Something I could always be proud of.

Watching the race on TV, I wondered if someday I might be able to do it. The idea was massive but motivating. My brain went to work sketching a loose plan of possibilities and what-ifs.

Right away, I knew that this was a long game. I'd have to start slow and build over time, continuously re-evaluating my options and potential. But since I was no longer focused on my professional career, I needed a goal. Ironman just might be it.

It sounds dramatic, but I've often felt that triathlons saved my life. In the fall of 2011, after eight of the toughest months imaginable, I knew things had to change. I had been tracking my pain and doing very little else. The drugs, the treatments. None of it worked. The only time I'd found any relief was when I was engaged in some kind of exercise or race.

I knew I had to set goals for myself and accomplish them. That was my old way of being; that was how I had achieved my quality of life before my accident and how I accelerated my recovery before 2011. I'd tell people I was going to do something that sounded crazy, like bike to Niagara Falls or do my first paratriathlon. And then I'd go out and do it, just to prove that I could. The bigger the goal, the more motivated I was to achieve it. After all the crap related to my spinal cord injury and being unable to solve my nerve pain challenges, I found myself at a point in my life where I needed to dream big. And I certainly thought the Ironman fit the bill. But I also knew I had to be smart about it.

My reputation for being a guy who does what he says is something I was proud of and wanted to preserve. So I wasn't in a rush to proclaim to the world that I was going to do a full Ironman. As overwhelmingly positive as my first Olympic distance triathlon had been, it was only 50.5 km long. To achieve 226 km in one day would be exponentially more difficult. I had a long way to go to hope to ever complete a full Ironman. I had a feeling I knew the scope of this goal and how big it was. So while in my mind I had decided that it was possible and I could do it, I held back from sharing this goal with the world. It was mine, and it was brewing inside of me. Instinctively, I knew that being smart meant breaking the uber goal into smaller ones. These smaller goals I could tell people about and get busy working on achieving.

Those first couple of years after the accident, I had thrown myself into training and competition in an all-consuming way. Starting from nothing, progress was immediate. I was almost always the only para-athlete when I raced. I was my only competition. Moving forward with the goal of doing a full Ironman, I'd need to be careful not to injure myself and make my disability even worse. I also knew that competing in international races meant that I wouldn't be alone out there. In addition to the race, I would have to steel myself to be prepared to race other athletes with similar disabilities.

My family doctor often told me that I was the most active patient she had and that maybe I should slow down. She commented that the healthcare system was proficient at replacing worn-out hips and knees but wasn't so effective at replacing worn-out shoulders, arms, hands, etc. The upper body wasn't designed to move you great distances on its own, and certainly not at heart rate threshold speeds. To avoid injury while getting stronger, I needed to make sure I left enough recovery time between workout days. And I needed to balance all the other responsibilities in my life as well: being a good husband and dad and not going overboard with other projects I did on the side, like the occasional public speaking engagement or mentoring. For an all-or-nothing kind of guy, ensuring I didn't overtrain would prove to be another significant goal to achieve.

At the beginning of 2012, I committed myself to my goal of doing an Ironman 70.3, also known as a Half Ironman, as it's half the distance (70.3 miles, or 113 km) of the full one, and I announced it to the world. This time, I was going to do it the right way. I was going to find a coach and work on my swimming. I was going to keep doing other competitions to build up my endurance. And my family and friends were going to be there at my side.

Rich agreed to train for and race the Half Ironman with me. He had done handcycling and wheelchair races before, but he had never done anything like the distance of an Ironman 70.3. Even more exciting, Sabrina was going to join us as well. She had gotten into triathlon when I was off in 2011, and after a couple of solid races, she was hooked. Like me, Sabrina was driven to challenge herself and to push her body beyond its comfort zone. We loved doing things like this together, such as the half-marathon we did in 2008. So, it made perfect sense that if one of us was going to sacrifice, suffer, and hopefully succeed, that, once again, we would do all of that together. With both of our girls now in school full time, we could even do a lot of our training together during the week. The drive and the opportunity were there... This was going to be awesome.

There's a joke in the triathlon community that triathletes have the unique distinction of being able to suck at three different sports, all at the same time. I think it's funny because it's true. The training required to swim, bike, and run multiple times a week at increasing distances, durations and intensities is exhausting. Add to that being a parent, working, managing a house, and maintaining friendships and the challenge of doing everything well can become overwhelming. To get really good at any one specific sport is ambitious, let alone three.

I know a few successful people who own and run large businesses and race Ironmans. They're typically in bed by ten and up around five. They find a way to get it done, and I'm always so impressed and inspired by seeing them do it all and doing most, if not all of it, well.

For me, I had the additional challenge of doing everything with my arms. I knew I was lucky that I could take a break from work to focus on sports. But training for an Ironman while having to deal with neuropathic pain weighed on me both physically and mentally.

When it came to my swim training, the time in the water was the easy part. The logistics before and after the swim were as much, if not more, difficult and taxing than pulling myself through the water. Swimming was hard.

I couldn't just grab my bag and go for a swim. A trip to the pool involved multiple transfers, lots of planning, and, ideally, some specialized equipment. For instance, I'd usually use the washroom at home to ensure I was empty, then drive to the fitness club, change down to my swimming shorts and head to the pool. Once on the deck, I'd test to see if the chairlift was working that day. If it wasn't, I had to decide if I was going to get in and worry about finding a way out of the pool and into my wheelchair when I finished my set or just not swim. Most of the time, I sucked it up and got my swim workout in. But on the days when I'd rather not swim at all, a broken chairlift meant that I didn't have to get wet and could instead spend extra time in the weight room.

If the chairlift was working, I'd lay my wetsuit pants on the pool deck and transfer out of my wheelchair to the ground. I'd zip up my custom pants along the side of each leg and then roll into the pool to start my swim. A typical swim would be 2 to 3 km of drills, exercises, and endurance.

After swimming for an hour or so, I'd remove my wetsuit pants in the pool, get in the chairlift or find a couple of guys to help pull me out of the pool, and then hit the showers. It wasn't uncommon to have to wait to take a shower because the one accessible shower stall was frequently occupied. Never mind that there were nine other normal shower stalls empty, which I pointed out to the person pissing me off. Once he finished or relocated, I'd transfer to the shower bench, shower, transfer back into my chair, dry myself off as best I could, get dressed while in my chair, transfer back into my car, and then head home. The one hour of swim training took about three-and-a-half hours out of my day. And when I got home, I'd probably have a bike ride or run session that I would feel compelled to do as well. I had to train my body and mind to learn that after swimming, there was still more work to be done. It was exhausting.

Bike training days were a little less complicated and involved. But whether I rode in the basement on the trainer or rode outside of my home, after most bike sessions, I'd do a run in my racing chair. As I worked towards getting ready to qualify, the training time on my watch ranged from six to thirteen hours a week depending on intensity and the phase of training I was in. When you added all the prep time and recovery, the number of hours focused on just triathlon was always over 30. Beyond triathlon, everything I was doing outside of sports also required the use of my arms, so I was tired and sore most of the time. But I was happy. I had a big goal to focus on, and I was doing it. I had something meaningful to chase, and I was making progress.

The Half Ironman is a steppingstone between the Olympic distance triathlon and a full Ironman distance race, like the one held in Kona. If I could do the Half Ironman quickly and consistently, I could then attempt a full, and one day maybe even try to qualify for the Ironman World Championships.

Once you've made the decision and commitment to train and race for a specific distance, the immediate next challenge as a wheelchair athlete is to find a race that is accessible (enough) and has welcoming organizers. Only a limited number of the Ironman branded races are accessible. On most courses, there's a set of steps, gravel, or grass on the run portion that makes advancing in the racing wheelchair dangerous, if not near impossible.

If you're an able-bodied triathlete, a good way to evaluate the accessibility of the run course is to consider whether you could ride your racing bicycle on it without having to get off and walk at any point. If you can't, then it's not likely a wheelchair athlete can complete the course without assistance. Even if there are volunteers waiting to help me over an obstacle, it's a barrier that other athletes don't have to face. And I'm at the mercy of the volunteers being ready, willing, and able.

Fortunately, in Ontario, the Multisport Canada Triathlon Series hosts a race that is only an hour from my home. It's flat, it's fast, and it's accessible enough. And the most important thing: the owner and his team welcome paratriathletes.

The Welland Half Ironman took place at the end of June. It was not an official Ironman branded event, but it was the same idea. The swim distance was actually a little bit longer than the official Half Ironman. It was a 2 km swim, the bike course was 90 km, and the run was a half-marathon distance, 21.1 km. My first Olympic distance triathlon was about seeing if I could finish it. For the Welland Half, I wanted to race it.

I'd learned that I could get two volunteers to help me with my transitions—they're called handlers in parasports—and it was a lot better than having a fellow competitor take the time to help me fumble through them. The handlers would not only help me out of the water and into the transition area, but they would also help me remove my wetsuit, get me in the handcycle, and then be there to scoop me up out of the handcycle and into the bucket of the racing chair. With handlers, I'd save a lot of energy and, more importantly, time.

Immersing myself in the world of triathlon, I quickly learned that sometimes you need to slow down to go faster. With something like an Ironman, or even a Half, it's not about the sprint. It's about endurance. At the gym or on our training bike rides at home, we focused on low heart rate miles. Lots and lots of miles. Longer distance triathlons are about training your body to maintain a solid pace for hours and hours without burning out.

I've always known the value of a good coach. In preparation for the Half Ironman, I began working with a young Pro Ironman Triathlete named Tyler. He saw me struggling in the LA Fitness pool one day and gave me some pointers. The guy was ripped and flew through the water, so I figured he might have some good advice to give.

While he was the first coach I had, I'd have the opportunity to work with a few others over the years. I had some great ones, most of whom I remain friends with today. These experts all had their strengths and quirks, but the one thing that none of my coaches had was specialized knowledge of para-sports. The mechanics of para-swimming, handcycling, and pushing a racing chair were totally foreign to them and me. But we were all eager to experiment and learn. To accelerate the learning process, I reached out to other para-athletes around the world who excelled in their sports and competed in the races I was interested in racing.

June came quickly. Before we knew it, it was race day. Sabrina, Rich, and I organized our equipment in transition and headed down to the water to begin our first Half Ironman distance race.

Swim starts can be chaotic. It's scary when the starting pistol is fired and everyone starts thrashing their arms at the same time. Competitors have been known to climb on top of others or kick them as they go by. You like to believe it's by accident, but I'm not so sure it always is.

Because my legs are zipped together in my wetsuit and I can't kick my feet, most swimmers don't see me. Worried about getting swum over or getting crushed, I hugged the edge of the water on the way out. That would also limit the impact of the current I was swimming against, and it helped to keep my heart rate as low as possible for the duration of the swim. I didn't want to use up all my energy in the water. Keeping my pace steady and avoiding any misadventures, I was able to complete the swim in a respectable time—not fast, but I wasn't last. And I was ahead of Rich.

The bike ride was very flat and fast, and I averaged over 28 km/h. It felt like I was hitting my stride. The run proved to be a bit more of a challenge, though. I was tired but still wanted to go hard. This was made even harder by the realization that I had messed up my nutrition by not drinking enough fluids on the bike. My stomach was upset, and I constantly felt like I would throw up.

Around the 8 km mark of the run, my arms started knotting up. By the 16 km mark, everything in my upper body started to go. My shoulders, my back, my arms—it was starting to seize. If I locked up completely, my race would be over.

The run was an out-and-back course. After the turnaround, I saw Rich. He was hurting, too. Knowing how strong, experienced, and competitive he was, I forced myself to block out the pain and push on with everything I had. I powered through to the finish in a time of 5:22:15. I was thrilled with my time and the race overall. I got it done. I used up every last ounce of energy I had to give, and I became the first-ever wheelchair athlete to finish this race.

Sabrina was also pleased with her accomplishment. I think Rich was, too, though I knew he didn't like coming in second place to me. He had beaten me in every other race we had prior to that day, so I felt like I had finally proven myself to him as a serious competitor.

While I was happy with how it had gone, I immediately went about identifying ways to improve. I felt one step closer to being able to complete a full Ironman. And I was very motivated to continue my training.

The summer of 2012 was special. The year before, we had purchased a small cottage in the Kawarthas, and we were going to move up there for the summer. After breaking my back, I could no longer get into the camping trailer that we loved so much. We sold the trailer in 2009, and I cried as the new owner drove it away. Finding this lake-front cottage on a lot that was flat from the driveway to the dock and only two hours away from home felt like winning the lottery. It was a very special purchase that we stretched ourselves to make, but we knew it would be the place where many new memories would be made. It was also the best place to conduct our triathlon training.

Triathlon wasn't the only thing that Sabrina and I were doing together in 2012. While the first couple of years following my accident we had worked on improving our physical intimacy, our success rate wasn't terribly impressive. By 2012, however, something clicked. We finally found our intimacy groove again. Maybe all the experimenting was starting to pay off, maybe it was a newfound confidence in my body that I had acquired, or maybe it was something with Sabrina. I don't know exactly why, but I do know that in the area of intimacy, we found a new happy place where we could enjoy and celebrate that part of our relationship again. I knew that it would never be as good as it was before my accident, but with the right attitude and a patient and curious approach, we were connecting again.

Living at the cottage for two months was simply the best. I loved waking up on the lake every day. Sabrina and I were in the best shape of our lives and felt blessed in many ways. Having finished strong in Welland, the question became what to do next. My dream was still the Ironman World Championship, but there was still a lot to do to get there.

Fortunately, I wasn't alone in wanting to push the limits of what was possible. Sabrina also felt great with her Welland finish and wanted more. As the summer of 2012 came to an end, we found ourselves dreaming and strategizing about what we might be able to accomplish in 2013.

When I was still able-bodied, I marvelled how anyone might be able to do an Ironman and was in awe of those I met who had actually completed one. Now, many years older and me being paraplegic, here we were getting excited about the idea of completing the full Ironman ourselves.

Strategically, we knew that it would be wise to complete at least one more Half Ironman race before attempting the full. Riding a high from our recent accomplishment, we couldn't wait until next June to race Welland again. That wait would have been too difficult. We needed the rush of the finish line before then. And we trusted that the more Half Ironman finishes we could complete before attempting a full, the greater the chance that we'd be successful. Combing the Ironman website for race options, we decided on and registered for Ironman 70.3 Oceanside, California, taking place at the end of March.

The next task was to find and register for a full Ironman that satisfied all of our requirements before it sold out. Louisville, Kentucky, was the one. It took place at the end of summer, so we had all of July and most of August to train for the longer distance. Louisville was only one long day's drive away, so we could turn this into a family holiday with the girls before they started back at school, and it was accessible (enough). Even though my research showed that Louisville was known to be one of the tougher Ironman races to do because of the crazy heat and a lot of climbing on the bike course, we were stoked.

Just registering for Louisville got my heart racing with excitement. When I finished, Sabrina asked me to sign her up too. "No way," I said. "If you want to do a full Ironman, you need to be the one to commit."

Even though I was thrilled that we were going to do this together, I knew the importance of us individually making the decision and commitment. This wasn't going to be easy, and the last thing I wanted was the potential of it coming up at some later time that I was the one that signed her up to suffer. Sabrina understood and registered that same day. The next 12 months were going to be something else.

During the fall and winter, we trained no less than five days a week at the fitness club doing weights and swimming, outside when the weather cooperated, and in the basement on trainers when it didn't. We did around half of the workouts together while the girls were in school or when they had something at home to keep them occupied. Before we knew it, it was March of 2013, and we were flying down to L.A. We stayed in Oceanside near the race start crammed into the official race hotel, which unfortunately was rather run down and dirty. The good thing about a less than comfortable hotel room was that we spent most of our time outside of it, checking out the sights and the racecourse. Oceanside is beautiful.

On race morning, around 5:30, Amir arrived at our hotel from L.A. to help us pack the minivan and get us and all our gear to the starting line. Once our bikes were sorted, we got into our wetsuits. My group started before Sabrina's, so we kissed and wished each other good luck before I headed down to the water. The ocean was freezing! Around 60 degrees. When my face touched the water, it literally took my breath away. I knew this reaction was an innate biological reflex, but it still surprised me.

At the sound of the starter's gun, I went out hard and tucked in behind a large group of able-bodied swimmers. I swam as hard as I could, partly to stay in the draft and give myself the best swim time possible, but also to try and generate some warmth in my body. My face was numb, and I knew that wasn't going to change. But I wanted my arms to at least loosen up a little. When I got to the swim exit, I got into my wheelchair with Amir's help and pushed into transition where my handcycle was waiting. Getting there, I was happy to see that I was currently leading the handcycle division. I wasn't alone here in Oceanside, which was a nice surprise. Ricky James was racing today. He was the kid I saw on TV five years before that inspired me to dream of doing an Ironman someday, and he just happens to be from Oceanside. My race was going well on many levels.

Out on the bike, it was the first time racing my new Carbonbike handcycle, and I worked hard at getting the power into the cranks just like I trained. The Oceanside bike course goes up and over a mountain. As strong as I felt on the handcycle back home in the basement on the trainer, I was quickly reminded that elevation and wind are two factors of riding outside that can't be underestimated. These factors are difficult to replicate when training indoors all winter. I was going slower than I had hoped. But I held the effort that I thought would be hard for Ricky to catch. And at the end of the 90 km, I continued to hold the lead on him.

During the bike segment, however, I had been passed by Sabrina. In triathlons, athletes with a disability are typically some of the first athletes to start the race to give us as much time as possible before the course had to be closed. This meant I usually had a head-start on Sabrina. And because we usually swam at a similar pace, but she cycled slightly faster than me, the entire time I was working hard to finish the bike course as quickly as I could, I was also looking forward to being caught and passed by my racing buddy. Sure enough, with 20 km left to go on the bike course, Sabrina passed me with a "Good job, babe!" shout-out. When that happened, I had even more motivation to go hard. I wasn't just trying to stay ahead of Ricky, but I was chasing my wife. *How awesome is this?* I thought to myself, smiling inside and out.

Within the first 5 km of the run portion of the race, I found myself trapped behind runners clogging the six-foot-wide running path that ran along the road. Even though most of the athletes were on the run portion of the triathlon, there were still cyclists coming towards us on the way to the transition area. In the racing chair, I can typically wheel twice as fast as the average able-bodied athlete can run. While I'm typically slower on the swim and the bike, the run is where I can usually improve my overall time and placement. Trying to get past the runners and up to speed, I yelled as loudly as I could, "Wheelchair on the left!" over and over, but no one heard me. Or, if they did, they didn't think to look behind them and move to the right.

After a few kilometres of this, I began to get really frustrated. It was then that Ricky flew by me on the road in his racing wheelchair, going head-on against the remaining athletes finishing the bike. *SHIT, there's goes the lead,* I thought to myself. *Okay... new rules, I guess.* I steered out of the running path and onto the road to try and chase him down.

At the 20 km mark of the run, I continued to have Ricky in my sights. However, I was starting to feel the fatigue of racing 100 kilometres so far and getting frustrated at runners that darted in front of my racing chair, requiring me to take evasive maneuvers to avoid hitting them. The advantage of this out-and-back looping run course was that I also got to catch and pass Sabrina a few times during the run. Seeing her running strong and knowing she was going to finish gave me a boost of adrenaline to try and catch Ricky, but after increasing my pace for 100 metres or so, the muscles in my arms started knotting up, and I had to ease off. While I was doing great, I didn't have fitness, strength, or maybe even the confidence needed to catch Ricky. That was okay.

The win wasn't terribly important to me; the big picture was. I was thrilled to be in California, racing with Sabrina and getting stronger and faster with every kilometre. I finished in a time of 6:05:46. Sabrina wasn't far behind me and came into the finish strong and smiling (as always). We had just done our first officially branded Ironman 70.3. We were exhausted but over-the-moon happy.

Back home in Ontario, spring was starting to arrive, and after a couple weeks of recovering from our travels and the Oceanside race, we began training outside again. We still had the Welland Half Ironman distance to race again in June, but all of our focus was on getting ready for the full Ironman in Louisville on August 25th.

Welland came quickly, and I was confident that I would crush my previous time from the year before. I was in the best shape of my life, and I had this new handcycle that was lighter and more aerodynamic than the one I used before. The previous year, I finished in 5:22:15. This year, I was aiming for sub-five-hours.

The swim was four minutes faster than last year's. On the bike, I knew I needed to be under three hours for the 90 km to achieve my goal for today but came up short. Even though I was stronger and on a better bike, the conditions on this day were much tougher than in 2012. The wind was constant, and the temperature was well into the 40s (Celsius) with the humidex. My increased effort over the previous year was not translating into a much faster pace. I started this race expecting to crush the bike course but was humbled and learned a very important lesson. Specifically, even if you're racing a course that you've completed before, don't assume that it's going to be the same experience. Challenging weather and other factors like not having a friend to chase or chase you makes a huge difference to your experience, and consequently, your results. Rich didn't sign up for the race again in 2013, so I didn't have my good friend to motivate me. I completed the bike course only three minutes faster and the run course only 30 seconds faster. Even though I set a new wheelchair athlete course record of 5:13:57, I didn't break the five-hour target I was hoping for.

In the racing wheelchair, travelling almost 20 km/h, the speed of the wind passing over me helps to cool my body. Sabrina didn't have this advantage. The entire run, she braved the distance and the heat (along with all the other athletes). Her time doing this race was a little slower than the year before, but once again, she proved how tough she was. When Sabrina set her mind to doing something, no matter how hard it gets or how much pain she has to suffer through, she never quits. She's tough.

At the end of the day, we went home a little battered and beat up. But we each had another medal for our wall and learned a number of well-earned lessons.

Back at the cottage for July and August, we juggled training and parenting. Chloe and Zara loved the cottage and were constantly in and out of the water, crafting, playing with the puppy, or training for their own kids' triathlon that would take place a week before Louisville. Sabrina and I would swim across the lake and back for our 1.8 km swim workouts and then play in the water with the girls until all of us were prunes and needing to dry out. The roads around the cottage were great for cycling, and each week our coach would add 10 to 15 km to the length of our long ride. Between a neighbour's daughter who took care of the girls and some lovely friends who helped us out, Chloe and Zara were patient as Sabrina and I continued to spend more and more time away from them training for the big race.

Twelve to 18 hours a week of training time became the norm that summer, with some rides taking as long as seven hours. We were tired but happy. The longest training practice day before starting the taper for Louisville involved a 3 km swim, 130 km bike, and 14 km run. It was the perfect test of doing all three disciplines on the same day, and I felt ready to start my taper. This training day was more difficult for Sabrina, as she had missed some training during the summer after contracting pneumonia. She was also nursing a bruised rib from a fall she took on the bike when she went off the edge of the pavement onto the gravel shoulder and lost the front end (ouch). Sabrina was less enthused about this particular training day. But, as I knew she would, she sucked up the pain and got it done. With a couple weeks of tapering ahead of us, we were feeling ready to head South and race.

Four days before the race, with our enclosed trailer filled with all our gear and luggage, we loaded up the SUV and started the drive to Louisville. We were thrilled that Sabrina's mom was coming with us, and our friends would meet us down there to provide support (and fun). Having a couple days to test our gear, check out the course and climatize to the heat was perfect. There's an energy to events like this, and it's hard to keep your excitement in check until race day. Having tapered for a few weeks, your body is revving with stored up energy. I erred on the side of doing less and saving every ounce of energy for race day. The anniversary of my accident was coming in October, and I really wanted to be able to prove to myself that I could go from breaking my back to Ironman in less than five years. As a bonus, I'd be the first Canadian paraplegic to complete this epic distance.

The race swim starts upriver from the transition area. Sabrina and I gave each other our pre-race kiss and wished each other a good race before I got a ride to the start from the organizers, and Sabrina started the long walk with all the other athletes. At 6:50 AM, they dropped us handcyclists in the water, and we started our swim 800 metres upstream in the Ohio River against the current before turning around the island and heading downstream the rest of the way. There were four of us handcyclists racing today, including Ricky James.

The bridges that span over the river make sighting easier than a typical race, but the pollution in the water is disgusting and distracting. I tried to focus on the current helping me most of the way and was careful not to drink any of the filth. I finished the swim in 1:26:25. I was in second place behind Ricky and thrilled to get on the bike. I knew Ricky wouldn't allow a repeat of Oceanside. Being experienced at this distance, he had the knowledge and confidence to go hard and win the day.

Like the Half Ironman races I had done before, I held to my target power number for the bike that I knew I could maintain all day. The two other handcyclists that finished the swim after me eventually passed me on the 180 km bike course. But I was okay with that; I let them go. I knew today was going to be a long day, and my goal was to finish, not to win. After a couple hours of cycling, Sabrina passed me on the bike as well. I was so proud of her for being here and proud of us as a couple. We were doing it.

After cycling for eight hours and 18 minutes, I rolled into transition. One of the handcyclists that had passed me earlier was taking his time getting himself organized and into his racing chair. I was psyched to start the run and began the last discipline in third place, feeling strong.

Exiting the transition area to start the run, Chloe, Zara, and my mother-in-law were there to cheer us on. Chloe was holding a neon yellow sign that read *ROB ROCKS!* with other shout-outs all around it like *#1 Dad, Keep Pushing, We (heart) you!* and *Go Super Dad.* Not to be outdone, Zara held a sign that read *Run like you stole something!* complete with an illustration of a bag of money and a smiley face. Classic Zara.

The marathon in Louisville is the opposite of Oceanside. It's flat and very fast. Most of the course takes place on a four-lane road that provided a lot of space for me to weave in and out of the runners while maintaining speed. The run course is two laps, so for the first, I held my power in check to ensure I wouldn't blow up and I'd be able to complete this race. Not long after starting the run, I passed Sabrina, and we cheered each other on. As I was nearing the finish of the first lap, I also passed the handcyclist that was in second place. I noticed he had gotten a flat tire. But with race organizers helping him to fix it, I didn't stop to chat.

On my second lap, I waited until I had 12 km to go before pushing as hard as I could. Summoning up every last watt of energy, I hit the rims hard and crossed the finish line in 12:32:54. After the longest racing swim and bike of my life, I set a new personal best for my marathon, in a time of 2:32:52.

Chloe, Zara, my mother-in-law, and friends were at the finish line to cheer me in. What a day! What a race! I just did the full Ironman with my arms. Anything IS possible. After pounding back a few litres of fluid, I got out of my racing chair and into my day chair. The girls went back with their Nani for a rest at the hotel. They'd come back in a couple of hours to cheer Sabrina in.

Refreshing the app on our phones every few minutes, we followed Sabrina's progress on the run and were waiting for her when she came running into the finishing chute. I'd never heard Chloe and Zara cheer so loudly in my life. It was late, and they had had a long day in the sunshine. In her bright pink tri-kit, Sabrina came running through the finish line with an even brighter smile than any race before. Now the day was perfect! Finishing in 14:54:44. Her first full Ironman, completed in less than 15 hours! We were all so proud and happy for her. For us. What an accomplishment.

Back at home with the girls in school, Sabrina and I rested and recounted the craziness of the last 15 months. Having been consumed with such a large goal for so long, there was definitely a hole in our lives that I felt uneasy with. For Sabrina, she had gone from a runner to an Ironman triathlete in a span of three short years. She had accomplished this massive goal. She was done. The thought of signing up for another full one was not a priority.

But for me, I was in a different place. My ultimate goal was still to race at the Ironman World Championships in Hawaii. Louisville was a serious accomplishment, but it was also just another rung on the ladder to one of the world's most prestigious races. I wanted Kona badly, but this was a quest that I was going to have to continue on my own.

Everyone's road to Kona is difficult, and I suspect most athletes' journeys are full of trials and tribulations. Every race start brings a mix of excitement and fear. Every swim, bike, and run has its own unique character that reveals something to you that you didn't know, expect, or remember. And there's always the possibility that something will go wrong and result in a serious injury. After Louisville, 2014 was filled with all sorts of different races. Each of them taught me at least one lesson that would help me with the next; I was growing my knowledge and experience over time.

My personal list of lessons learned is long and includes a wide array of obstacles that most people wouldn't even think about. From negotiating with the race organizers so that I can park my truck close to the starting line to limit the amount of energy I need to expend getting all of my gear to the race start, to figuring out how and when I'm going to empty my bladder during the race without having to stop. From learning to avoid any swimmers in front of you doing whip-kicks (so you don't get kicked in the face, again), to learning how to get around runners who take up the entire path or street and are oblivious to you yelling, "Wheelchair on your left!" Every race taught me something, and I made sure to remember those lessons before the start of the next. Making a mistake once was understandable; making the same mistake twice was unforgivable.

With some cycling podiums, three Half Ironman distances and one full Ironman behind me, every mile and race gave me a little more confidence to begin the specific task of trying to qualify for Kona. Knowing I'd be going up against some of the best in the world, I had to be sure I was ready.

In theory, anyone can sign up for an official Ironman event. But for paratriathletes—or "handcyclists," as we're referred to in official Ironman documentation—there are a limited number of full and Half Ironman races we're allowed to compete in. The reasons for this vary. Mostly, it has to do with the accessibility of the course, the accessibility of the host city (or country), or the organizers' comfort at having athletes with a disability participate in their race for any number of personal (and not always accurate) reasons.

To race at the World Championships, athletes need to qualify by completing and placing very high, or winning, their category in an official Ironman event. There are a few exceptions for athletes to qualify through a lottery because of their celebrity or by being featured and followed for having an especially inspirational story. But none of those were available to me. I was going to do the work and qualify the old-fashioned way.

For able-bodied athletes, there are over 20 different full Ironman races each year where they can attempt to earn their ticket to Kona. For handcyclists, there are only three half Ironman races, where a total of four male handcycling tickets can be won.

Essentially, I'd need to win the handcycling division in Texas or Australia or come first or second for the remaining two spots in Luxembourg. Coming from Canada, I had no choice but to go abroad to try and qualify.

Australia was too far to be practical. Texas was the closest, but Luxembourg had only a few athletes show up in 2014, and they had finishing times that were similar or longer than my Welland races. So I thought I'd have a reasonable chance to beat athletes competing in Europe for the spot. Luxembourg Ironman 70.3 in 2015 was my goal, but there was a lot to do before I got on a plane.

As June 2015 approached, I felt ready for Luxembourg. I had trained hard, attended a winter training camp in Florida, found and began working seriously with a new primary coach, and even received some swim coaching from a friend. On top of that, I did my usual reaching out to and receiving advice from the growing community of wheelchair athletes that I knew. I was as ready as I would ever be. It was time to make the big push to Luxembourg and then, hopefully, to Kona.

After a long flight to Germany and a drive to Luxembourg, Sabrina and I settled into our hotel and got the lay of the land. My nephew, Zoe, and his fiancée, Nina, came from Germany to spend time together and help me with the race. When I ventured over to the race registration, I was shocked to learn that, unlike the previous year, I was one of seven handcylists competing. Not only that, but I would be up against a past Ironman World Championships record holder. Fuck.

I introduced myself to my competitors, and they were mostly friendly and sociable. But when the race started, they all meant business. Another challenge that I had to face in this race was doing it without Sabrina. This would be the first race in a long time that I didn't have my racing buddy pushing me to go faster on the bike and giving me the motivation to go faster on the run to catch her before the finish. While I knew she would be the loudest fan cheering me on from the side of the road, I was going to miss her on course.

I had the race of my life. It was one of the most beautiful courses I'd ever raced, pushing along the Mosel River, through vineyards, and even cobblestone villages with old men smoking cigarettes yelling, "*Allez, allez, allez!*" at me. But I came in fourth. The three guys ahead of me were seasoned athletes, and I was the newbie. I didn't get the spot to go to Kona, and I was pretty upset about it. This wasn't part of my plan.

Sabrina and I made the most of our remaining few days in Europe. We went cycling, saw the sights, and soaked up the culture. It was a nice treat to have Sabrina all to myself for a change, and I loved just being with her and experiencing new places and things. The fact that we were in such a picturesque and storied part of Europe was a bonus. The romance of the area and experience was infectious and inspiring.

Back home, I took some time to recover from the race, the travelling, and my disappointment. We packed up and moved to the cottage for the summer again. I was sad that I wasn't going to Kona.

Speaking with my primary coach, we went over the race and the training I did leading into it. She suggested we do an exercise where we list the things that we could have done differently or that we just didn't do to prepare for Luxembourg. This was supposed to give me focus for the qualifier next year, assuming I wanted to keep going. Rather than inspire me, though, this list just made me angry.

If she knew things that I should have been doing but didn't tell me about them, or push me to try them, then she wasn't the best coach for me. I had basically committed the better part of my waking hours to this goal and would do whatever I had to do to accomplish it. I needed a coach that was going to be as committed as me. Someone who was proactive and got in front of any issues or weaknesses I had so that we could problem-solve them before race day. We parted on friendly terms, and I decided I was going to continue with my goal of getting to Kona, but with a different coach.

The triathlon training camp I attended in Florida during the winter of 2015 was excellent. Not only were the coaches all highly experienced racers and trainers, but their athletes were incredibly kind, hardworking, helpful, and successful. Many of Canada's fastest triathletes were coming from this team, so it made perfect sense to me that I should reach out to them and see if one of the coaches that helped me at the camp would be interested in helping me get to Kona. Luckily, there was interest, and I started working with my new coach right away to get me back on track. We agreed that I'd do things differently for the qualifier in June 2016 in Texas.

I'd worked hard leading into Luxembourg. But I took things to an entirely new level for my second chance to qualify. I trained my ass off. For the nine months leading to Texas, I didn't miss more than a handful of the workouts that my new coach put in my schedule. I was focused and determined because I knew that if I didn't qualify for Kona this time, I probably never would. And I didn't want to live with the regret of knowing that there were things I could have done but didn't. I was going to give it my all and take one last shot at getting to the Big Dance.

My nephew Callum joined me on the journey to Texas, which was awesome. He and my good friend's brother-in-law, who lives in Lubbock, were my handlers for the race.

In 2015, just a couple of guys showed up in Texas for the two spots that were available that year. In 2016, there were seven guys racing for one ticket to Kona. I recognized some of the other racers from previous races, like Louisville. One of the other athletes was someone I knew about but hadn't met yet. His name is Scot, and he had just gotten back from Luxembourg, where he won the race and already earned his ticket to Kona. It was incredible to think he could do two Half Ironman races on back-to-back weekends, on two different continents. But all I could do was stay focused and push hard, and hope that I wanted it more than anyone else did.

I came out of the water in fourth, had the strongest bike of all the handcyclists and caught the leader in transition. It was Scot, who, because he had qualified for Kona in Luxembourg, wouldn't need the Kona ticket up for grabs in Texas. I chased Scot the entire run, not concerned with passing him for first place and potentially risking blowing up or crashing. Rather, I was focused solely on ensuring that I was not caught by one of the guys behind me.

At the end of that race, I was mentally and physically exhausted not only from the race itself but from the years of training that had led up to it. I had pushed my body and mind to their limits while struggling with neuropathic pain. But I had done it. When I rolled over the finish line, I knew I'd had a great race. I had qualified for Kona.

I was thrilled and a little scared. I had accomplished my goal of qualifying, but now I had only three months to train my body to go twice the distance I had just done. The full Ironman lay ahead of me, but that could wait until I was home. That night, Callum and I would celebrate in Texas.

But first, I needed to call Sabrina: "Baby! We're going to Hawaii!"

Chapter 10
The Ironman World Championships

The President's Award for Outstanding Achievement that I was awarded from Microsoft during the summer of 2008 brought recognition and a trip to Hawaii for my partner and me. Scheduled for November, I was so excited knowing I'd get time away with Sabrina in one of the most beautiful places in the world. But the accident had foiled that trip. I broke my back on October 5th. So, in addition to losing so much related to my health and mobility, I lost the opportunity to reward Sabrina and myself for all of our hard work and dedication to my career. I had so been looking forward to that trip, and not being able to go had added immensely to my sadness and frustration.

In 2009, we began taking the odd night away from home and even tried some little vacations. At first, they were basically experiments to see what I could do and what we would enjoy as a young family. The first bigger trips that involved flying were on two separate Caribbean cruises. They were fine, but the motion sickness that stayed with Sabrina for a few weeks after each trip discouraged us from doing more of them.

By 2012, we were getting more adventurous. And with the exception of a couple all-inclusive resort-type vacations, we started focusing on what we liked to call "race-cations." A trip that included a race alongside the sightseeing.

We did the New York City Half-Marathon, the Bermuda Triangle Challenge, Oceanside, Louisville, Luxembourg, and Texas Half Ironman events. It was exhausting having to navigate airports, planes, rental cars, taxis, hotels, beaches, etc., especially when we had to bring all of our racing gear. But each trip was special in its own way, and all the race-cations included bringing back a finishing medal, and—for the trips that Chloe and Zara joined us on—they generated fond memories.

But going to Kona meant something different. It was more than a race-cation. It meant getting back something very specific that I felt cheated out of because of my accident. Practically speaking, I could have gone to Hawaii on vacation with my girls at any point after I'd recovered enough to travel, but that would have been far less meaningful. Going to Kona to race the World Championships would be the pinnacle of accomplishment for me and something we could all experience, enjoy, and remember as a family. If I had needed extra motivation to qualify for and finish this race, I had it.

We arrived in Kona a week before race day. I felt lucky to have found and booked probably the last wheelchair-accessible condo anywhere near Kona. Because, of course, we didn't know we were going until the end of June when I qualified in Texas. And that was only three-and-a-half months before the World Championships. By the end of June, pretty much everything that you could book or rent, especially with an ocean view, was already taken.

The condo was a bit run down, but it was in a nice community. For sure, it was nothing like the accommodations that would have been provided by Microsoft. But we had a view of the ocean and a place to call our home for two weeks. It was, in its own way, perfect.

We had a week to prepare and adjust to the climate. And we jumped right into the Hawaiian experience, going on a snorkelling tour and to a luau our first days there. It was a dream trip come true. At the luau, the girls were adorned with leis and flowers in their hair as the entertainment treated us to a history of Hawaii through music, stories, and food. Yes, it was touristy. But we were tourists, happily soaking up every minute of it.

The following day, instead of me doing a swim workout on my own, we decided to do a "swim with dolphins" excursion. It was incredible. We went out on a boat, and the operators searched the coast for pods of dolphins. When we found one, they positioned the boat around 500 metres out in front of the dolphins, and we all got into the water, just in time to have the dolphins swim by us. We did this a few times. Chloe was almost 13 and Zara 10 and were very strong swimmers, which allowed us all to fully enjoy the experience. Overall, the tour was over rather quickly. But it was so special to be out in the ocean with these magical creatures.

On our way back to the condo, we stopped to check out the town of Kona. Sabrina purchased a gift shop ukulele and some snacks for the girls. Zara had started playing the ukulele back home and was a quick learner. She showed Chloe what she knew, and throughout our entire holiday, the sweet sounds of music and harmonies filled the air, supported by the background of waves crashing on the rocks beside our condo. Later in the week, we purchased a high-quality ukulele from a proper instrument store, and Sabrina posted a recording of them singing "Tonight You Belong to Me - Chloe & Zara" on YouTube. It was perfect.

It was an amazing experience to be there with Sabrina, Chloe, and Zara. Back at home, there were far fewer opportunities to spend quality time together. Chloe had been accepted to Canada's National Ballet School at the age of ten and had moved into a residence when she started grade six. She was one of only 25 grade six students from around the world invited to live, complete her academics, and study ballet at this prestigious school. To say we were proud of her would be an understatement. Her quiet confidence and perseverance made her shine. It was the perfect opportunity for her, even though we missed her dearly, as she spent most of the year at school and came home to be with us only on Saturday nights and holidays. Some of our family and friends told us they would never allow their child to move away from them at such a young age. Our response was simple. It wasn't about us.

As for Zara, she was equally driven, but her passion was ponies and horses. She cherished every opportunity she had to be at the barn with her mom. The barn was her happy place, and she often remarked that if there was a private school where she could ride as much as Chloe danced, she'd be there. Even with her at home, my time with Zara was limited by virtue of her diligent work ethic for academics and the hobbies that she'd take up and master, like knitting, sewing or ukulele, and of course, the all-important barn time. I tried not to be jealous by remembering that at least she slept in her own bed at night. And every morning I could wake to hearing her in the kitchen below our bedroom, making herself breakfast, caring for the cats, playing with the dogs, and organizing her lunch and snacks for the day. I always tried to get out of bed in time to kiss her goodbye before she headed out the door, and I would smile to myself with confidence that I had nothing to worry about with my baby. My little firecracker was a force of nature, and both my girls made me so very proud. I just hoped I was doing the same.

Every day in Hawaii, we made amazing memories that would last a lifetime. Swimming at the public beach with sea turtles, the ice-slushie-truck in the parking lot, the sunsets on our patio… We loved every moment and found lots of time to play, rest, and cuddle together. All the pain and struggle to get here was already worth it. I was happy.

Prior to race day, I also made a point of finding time to connect with some athletes that I'd reached out to for advice prior to qualifying. They were from all over the world, and I thought it was special that we could all meet face-to-face on the Big Island.

When race day came, we were up and out of the condo just after 4:00 AM. As we approached the bay, we saw the growing glow of the lights in and around the transition area peering out into the pitch-black sky. I was one of the first athletes to check in. Night turned into day as the sun slowly rose, replacing the calmness in the air with excitement and pre-race jitters. At times like these, the energy that surrounds you is palpable.

Thirty minutes before the pros started, helicopters began to circle. This is when you know that shit is about to get real. The Pro Men started, then Pro Women. I got my wetsuit on, and my handlers carried me into the water. I swam towards the start line and treaded water with the Age Group Women. I knew the other handcyclists were in the water as well, but I couldn't see them amongst the sea of pink swim caps. I was on my own, and the race was about to start. Time to focus.

A cannon fired to start the race. There were small swells stirred up by the breeze that made swimming in a straight line difficult. But it was beautiful. The water was crystal clear upwards of 100 feet deep, teeming with all sorts of marine life. I tucked behind a woman in a bright pink tri-suit, letting her do the sighting while I could get a draft. This was going to be the longest ocean swim I'd ever done in my life, and I had a long day ahead of me after that.

The goal for the swim was to get it done without using up too much energy. It went well, and after an hour and thirty-three minutes, I was swimming up to my waiting handlers. They pulled off my wetsuit pants, scooped me up out of the water, ran me through the freshwater showers to get the salt off my skin, and laid me into my handcycle.

By that point, transition was pretty much empty. There were 2,197 athletes ahead of me, including Jason and Scot on their handcycles. I got my helmet on and took a final spray of sunscreen, and then I started the bike. It felt good to be pedalling, and the enthusiasm of the spectators was like fuel to me. I think they were just as excited as us athletes from the way they hooted, hollered, and cheered us on. It was awesome.

On the bike, I tried to hold off on going too hard too early. That's tough with all the excitement and cheering. But while I wanted to make up time, I also needed to pace myself. I watched my power numbers closely and stayed close to optimal—just like I had trained. I had been warned not to get caught up in the temptation to push too hard in the city. The remaining handcyclist who finished the swim after me passed me 10 km into the bike, but I let him go. I'd stick to my race plan. I reminded myself that this was going to be the hardest bike ride of my life, so best to hold back a little.

On the Queen Ka'ahumanu Highway, the headwinds were strong. I could feel the momentum being sapped out of me from the tropical wind, which takes the heat from the asphalt and lava fields lining the highway and beats you down. It's not unlike that surprise rush of hot air you get when you're baking cookies and open the oven door. Except, this was constant.

Around the 30 km mark, I passed the handcyclist who had overtaken third place from me in town. And shortly after that, I passed Minda. Minda is amazing. The first female handcyclist to ever complete at Kona, she was going for her second finish.

Sixty kilometres in, and I had to acknowledge that this was an entirely new level of difficulty. As tough as training in cottage country back home in the Canadian summer was, it didn't compare to a Hawaiian island. In Ontario, training in 30-plus degree Celsius weather, I averaged a two-litre Camelbak of Eload, which is like Gatorade, over 90 km or three hours. But after 60 km of cycling the big island, my Camelbak was dry. Shit! I was thirsty, and there was nothing I could do but power on and grab a bottle or two of liquids at the next aid station.

A lot of the aid stations are on an uphill as it's easier to pass bottles to cyclists when they're climbing versus flying by at over 40 km/h. That's fine for able-bodied cyclists who can continue to pedal while they feast on their gels and fluids. For me, I had to stop pedalling and hold my brake so I wouldn't roll backwards as I grabbed a bottle and chugged as much of it as I could.

While I was stopped for hydration, I also put some more sunblock on my lips, which were starting to burn. I grabbed a spare bottle of Gatorade before the end of the aid station and tried to find a place to keep it on my bike. I didn't have bottle cages on my handcycle because I had planned on just using the Camelbak that I started with and one that I would pick up after the halfway point of Havi at the special needs station. But that was at around the 100 km mark. I still had a long way to go.

Stopping for a minute at aid stations on a 180 km bike ride should not be a big deal to an Ironman competitor. And I don't suspect it is for any of the able-bodied athletes. But for handcyclists, hills pose a particular challenge. The problem with stopping at all is that us handcyclists are held to the same time cut-offs as all the other athletes. So, if we don't make it to the turnaround in Hawi or other designated points along the route in time, our day is over, and we get driven back to the start line.

Watching my power, my average speed, and my time, I kept telling myself that I wouldn't fail, I couldn't fail, I was going to get this done. I reminded myself that I had prepared for this distance and these conditions and that if my mind told my body to do something, it wouldn't let me down.

After 63 km of cycling, you turn left onto Kawaihae-Mahukona Road. It starts with a steep downhill that goes by quickly, followed by almost 30 km of climbing to get to the turnaround point in Havi. The first 20 km have small downhill breaks, but the last 10 km are continuous climbing. All that against the hot wind with no shade to speak of.

This was it. If I could make it to the turnaround and beat the bike cut-off, I should be able to make up time coming down the mountain and finish the cycling portion in time. I pushed on climbing, focused on the next ten feet in front of me, and then the next.

I saw one of the handcyclists come screaming down the mountain on his way back to Kona, but it barely even registered with me. There was no time to think about that, so I just closed my eyes and focused on getting consistent power into the pedals.

After four-and-a-half hours of cycling, I reached the turnaround at Hawi, 95 km into the bike. Coming back down the mountain felt so good. The speed, the wind in my face—that was my reward for making the Hawi cut-off time. For a few moments, I was hitting over 65 km/h. But that only meant that the descent was over quickly. In practically no time at all, I was back to the grind.

And it was a grind. The unfortunate reality of Kona is that the winds often change direction in the afternoon. So, while I had the wind against me going out to Hawi, I also had the wind pushing against me on the way home.

As the hours continued to tick by, I did everything I could to stay focused. I thought about my girls standing in the hot sun waiting for me. I recounted all of the days riding hundreds of kilometres back home and always making it home. I remembered looking at my Training Peaks calendar and the sea of green—successfully completed—workouts that I had accomplished. I kept on the pedals and made sure to drink as much as I could. I had a total of 10 hours and 30 minutes from the start of the race (including my swim and transition) to complete the bike course, or my day would be over. I couldn't fail.

I pulled in at 9 hours, 56 minutes, and 45 seconds on the race clock. I had just cycled for 8 hours and 16 minutes. My skin was burned, my lips were fried and stinging. But I was one marathon away from conquering this epic race.

The transition area was full of bikes but no athletes. All the able-bodied athletes had come and gone. In fact, hundreds of athletes had already finished the entire race!

I was surprised to see the handcyclist that I passed on the bike course sitting in the transition area eating pizza. It took me a few seconds to register that the reason he wasn't still behind me on the bike course was that he didn't make the Hawi cut-off and was driven back to the start/finish.

When my handlers asked me if I wanted a slice of pizza, I was miffed. I was most likely on the verge of heat exhaustion, lying down on my bike, and they were offering me pizza?

Contemplating for a second what I had just accomplished, the tears started to flow. I gave myself 20 seconds to have that little release and then got my head back into the race. "Okay, Rob, you've just completed the Kona swim and bike! Now pull it together and finish this thing!" I told myself. I signalled to my handlers that I was ready, and they scooped me out of my handcycle and put me in my racing chair.

There was a little climb right out of the transition that I struggled up. I was a little dizzy from going so hard in the bike (on my back) all day to now being up high in my wheelchair, leaning forward. There were no crowds around transition anymore, but that was okay. After a couple of pushes, I heard the sweet sounds of Sabrina, Chloe, and Zara cheering me on. They walked beside me as I struggled to get up the first incline. Their cheers and excitement powered me onto a flat section, where I pulled away for the first stretch of the run course.

This first section goes out and comes back along the ocean. Around 3 km in, I hit my first set of rollers. I slowed to a crawl, but I was cheered up the hill by an Australian woman whose accent and choice of words made her sound like a sexy drill sergeant with the mouth of a trucker. She cursed that hill for me and got me up it with a smile.

As the daylight began to slowly fade, I hit the turnaround to come back towards town and my girls. With the sun setting into the ocean, the view was stunning. I took a mental picture. It was so beautiful. It was perfect.

As if racing on the Big Island of Hawaii wasn't enough of an incredible experience, the knowledge that I was getting close to accomplishing my goal made it all the more satisfying. At this stage of the race, there were other runners around me. It felt so good to be passing able-bodied athletes and getting back into the crowd that I had started with, even if I had to focus and dodge traffic. To my surprise, a lot of these athletes were either walking or running slowly. There was comfort in knowing I wasn't the only one suffering.

After that long bike ride, I knew I wasn't going to set any kind of a record this day. I knew how strong Jason and Scot were in the racing chair and that it was impossible for me to catch up to them. And feeling as though this might be my only time racing the World Championships, I decided to play the smart game of pushing at a slightly less aggressive pace. This would reduce the risks of me hitting a runner and ending both of our days. Or me hitting the point where my body would shut down from exhaustion, which would also end my day in a DNF (did not finish). I focused on trying to stay hydrated and consuming enough calories to get me to the finish.

Back in town, I turned right onto Palani Road and started my toughest climb of the entire race. The hill is so steep that many of the able-bodied athletes will just walk up it. For us wheelchair athletes, we needed to be careful not to tip over backwards. It's that steep.

I was so grateful that my girls were there to cheer me up the climb. The funny thing is that I couldn't look at them because I knew I'd start to cry. Instead, I focused just in front of my chair and grabbed the outside of my wheels for leverage. With each push, I moved another few inches up the hill. For 15 minutes, one push at a time, I slowly climbed.

Spectators came right up beside me and yelled inches from my face. "You've got this!" they said. "Push!" "Go, buddy, go!" Minda told me the day before, "The spectators won't let you fail on Palani." She was right.

Ten minutes into the climb and my girls were still beside me with their classic "GO, DADDY, GO!" chant. In addition to holding signs that they made, Zara had something new for this special race. She had acquired a mini cowbell which she diligently clanged for the entire hill. Right beside me. The entire hill! She was there.

Breaking my focus, I turned my head and as patiently as I could, especially considering my situation, and yelled, "Zara, no more cowbell!" The clanging stopped immediately, and Zara happily increased the volume of her "GO, DADDY, GO!" Within minutes I found myself cresting the hill and making my way back on the Queen K highway, into darkness this time. Thanks again, girls!

The highway has quite a bit of elevation to it. Driving a car, you might not notice. But it was very apparent pushing the chair. I made sure to take advantage of the downhills to get my speed up and recover a little, but I had to be careful. It was getting dark, and everyone was tired. It was easy to make a mistake that would be disastrous.

Around 14 km into the run, I was cruising down a hill and resting my neck, allowing my head to hang down. I followed the lines painted on the road passing beneath me. I should have been looking ahead to where my chair was going. Because all of a sudden, with no warning at all, I found myself thrust up into the air, on two wheels, on the verge of tipping over. What the fuck?!

I glanced back and saw what must have been a shuttered aid station by the side of the road, with all its tables stacked on the gravel beside the pavement amidst the tall grass. The ends of the tables, however, were sticking out into the bicycle lane ever so slightly, hidden by the tall grass beside the road and the darkness. I had just clipped that pile of tables and turned them into a ramp for my back wheel, causing me to nearly topple over. It scared the shit out of me, but it was a good reminder. The race wasn't over yet, and anything could happen.

I stayed focused on carrying on, down through the Energy Lab and back to the highway for the return to town. Turning down Palani Road, I held the brake to be safe and enjoyed the energy of the crowds and athletes cheering those of us who were still racing. The streets were glowing and alive. It was a dramatic and welcome contrast to the lonely miles in the pitch black of the highway among the lava fields.

Turning right onto Lahani Drive, I could hear the roar of the crowds and the announcer calling in the athletes. I got a burst of energy as I saw the red-carpeted finishing chute, lined with spectators five or more deep. All of them were screaming and cheering with their hands outstretched, wanting to give me a high-five as I passed. I tried to high-five as many people as I could while still pushing and maintaining some momentum. I was soaking this up.

As the finishing line approached, I looked up to see a ramp installed at the finish. It was steep, around ten feet long and four feet high! I put my head down and tried to get as much speed as possible before hitting the ramp. I got two feet from the top, and with my last ounce of energy, I muscled the push rims one last time to get over the line.

And then I heard Mike Reilly over the loudspeaker: "ROBERT BUREN, YOU ARE AN IRONMAN!" Holy shit! I did it! With a total time of 13:30:26.

To say I was a mix of emotions would be an understatement by great proportions. If I wasn't so dehydrated, I might have cried. But I was also overwhelmed with happiness and pride. I had to find my girls.

Before I was allowed to leave the finish area, I was intercepted by one of the volunteers who checked on athletes as they crossed the finish. He asked me to spit, but very little came out. So, the first stop would have to be the medical tent to get an IV.

On my way to the medical tent, one of my handlers came to congratulate me on second place. It turned out Scot had crashed his handcycle in town on a high-speed off-camber turn. Scot was in a no-passing zone, but a cyclist came alongside him mid-turn and surprised him. This caused him to lose control and roll the trike. He'd hurt his shoulder quite badly and tried to carry on, but he knew the challenge of the bike course and called it a day before leaving town. Scot had been another casualty of this epic challenge. The next day I learned from Zara that after the ambulance patched him up, Scot went back

What's Next

to the racecourse to cheer on the athletes still racing. I was incredibly impressed by his sportsmanship. What a classy guy.

In the medical tent, I was on a cot surrounded by athletes getting various types of treatment. I expected to get an IV, but the head doctor questioned if I really needed it or not. I think he was trying to save the Ironman Corporation thirty bucks. Asshole. I sipped on some Gatorade and waited for what felt like an hour. Fed up, I decided that if I wasn't going to get an IV, then I wanted to go and find my family. They let me go.

I went and found my girls, and we had a big celebration. Hugs and kisses, posing for photographs, the whole works. But just when we were about to pack my gear into the truck to head back to our condo, I started feeling faint. I put my head down on my lap and one of the medical volunteers saw me. Back to the medical tent I went, where they immediately got an IV line into me. My body started shaking, and I was totally out of it. All I could think of was *Fix me. Please, fix me!*

I had missed the hydration window while waiting for the IV the first time. Because my stomach was upset, and I assumed I'd be getting an IV when I first went to the medical tent, I hadn't pounded back the bottles of Gatorade like I should have. After two IVs and multiple vital checks, they loaded me into an ambulance and took me to the hospital. I really wanted to go back to the finish line and cheer on the last people getting in, but it was not going to happen.

At the hospital, they put me on more bags of IV and started their own battery of tests. They immediately worried that I had a condition where the body starts attacking the muscles, including the heart, in response to being overworked. They thought that they might have to fly me to another island where I could see a specialist. I just wanted them to fix me, and I was worried that I had pushed myself too hard and done lasting damage.

I spent a restless night in the hospital, but in the morning, the test results came back. It turned out I was just dangerously dehydrated and also suffering from a bladder infection, a common UTI. In retrospect, I was surprised I could do an Ironman while fighting a UTI. But I'm grateful I did. The hospital gave me some antibiotics to clear it up and said I would be fine.

Thankfully, I got to go to the awards ceremony later that evening. What an experience. I was up there on stage with some of the most amazing athletes in the world, and while my first goal of the race was to finish it, my secondary goal was to at least come in third so that I could be up there on that stage getting a medal. It was a very unexpected thrill to have placed second in my category.

I thought about the road that it took to get me on that stage. The blood, sweat, and tears. It was all worth it. Sabrina, Chloe, and Zara cheered me on one last time as I wheeled on stage to get my medal, bowl, and lei. It was an amazing night after a day of racing I'll never forget.

We still had a week on the island for sleeping and recovering. Although I moved a lot more slowly and gingerly than I had during our first week there, we still managed to do some sightseeing and a late-night swim with manta rays. The memories we made would last forever. The trip that we had missed out on years before had now not only happened with Sabrina but with our entire family.

And I had accomplished something that would forever be a defining achievement of my life. Before flying home, I started thinking about and designing what my M-Dot Ironman tattoo would look like. This accomplishment deserved some ink.

Chapter 11

Lessons Learned

After Kona, I needed a break. So, for more than a year, I stopped the intense swimming, biking, and running and had no plans for racing. I still did workouts to stay healthy and to help manage the pain, but I was seriously burnt out.

In addition to lacking motivation, or maybe contributing to a lack of motivation, I experienced what many athletes refer to as the "Post-Ironman Blues." I remember experiencing this a little after Louisville, but this time it was a lot worse. Having invested so much of my life into this one important goal and to have finally achieved it came at a cost. A significant void was created when I no longer spent the bulk of my time and energy focused on training 16+ hours a week and then trying to recover efficiently so I could train even more. Nor did I have the energy to define and start working towards the next goal.

It took many months to realize and come to terms with the reality that I had successfully completed a major goal in my life and that it was okay to slow down and enjoy that success. To feel okay with the idea that taking a well-deserved rest wasn't me being lazy or unmotivated. It was all about recovering.

In addition to recharging your batteries both physically and mentally following the completion of a big goal, the recovery window is also a good time to take stock of where your life is at. Slowing down to look back and to understand what exactly contributed to where you are now. Then gaining clarity on where you and your family are heading and asking why and if that's the best plan. That is so crucial to making the most of your life. Taking stock can be difficult and messy, especially if you're very critical about things. But I think it's a really important exercise that we all should do.

Before my accident, the only time I really slowed down to look at my life, reassess and regroup was when I was away from home on vacation. After the Ironman, I had time to identify what got me from breaking my back in the forest to the finish line in Kona. Even though I was home and not on vacation, my life wasn't all about training and preparing for the next workout. Doing this exercise is how I came up with four key lessons that I've learned since breaking my back.

I was speaking to younger audiences in universities when I first started sharing my lessons learned. I hoped that young people with so much of their lives ahead of them would find my discoveries relevant and helpful to defining and achieving their own goals. Oddly enough, even though these were my lessons and I was almost 50 years old, I realized that I continuously found value in reviewing them. Doing so helped to keep me focused and moving in the right direction. Consequently, it occurred to me these lessons might be valuable to anyone at any age or stage of life. There was certainly no harm in sharing.

The first lesson I've learned is to focus on what I can do, not on what I can't. This is a daily, if not hourly, task that drives my mood and motivation. It's not an automatic thing for me. Rather, it's a conscious task to constantly refocus my attention and the story I'm telling myself. Lots of self-talk takes place in my head: "I'm lucky I can still move my arms. I'm lucky I didn't suffer a brain injury. I'm lucky to be alive." Even many years after my accident, if I let my brain go to a place of focusing on what I've lost and stay there too long, it's a recipe for making myself miserable and someone that no one will want to be around.

The second lesson I've learned is to always have goals that I'm working towards. The goals can be small or big, but they should be achievable with enough hard work and maybe a little luck. I think the accomplishment of the Ironman is a great example of how an enormous goal can be broken down into smaller accomplishments along the way.

I didn't go from breaking my back to becoming an Ironman overnight. I started out learning how to get around my neighbourhood in my day chair. Then I learned how to ride a handcycle, building strength indoors on a trainer before heading outside to complete short 5 km rides. Next, I moved on to the racing chair and swimming. I kept the big goal in the back of my mind and focused on achieving smaller, more immediate goals that would ultimately contribute to and facilitate that larger objective.

With racing, I started out with short, single races in each discipline. Over time, I put them together to race a short triathlon. Success at this drove me to complete multiple Half Ironman races and, eventually, the full Ironman. Every finish line, in addition to giving me the satisfaction of completing a goal, immediately demanded of me, what next? Could I do that sport further, faster, or in a more challenging race?

I figured out what motivated me, which was always having a challenging goal to focus on and work towards. I also learned that this is what made me happiest.

One of the secrets to this second lesson learned was the value of measuring and tracking my progress over time. Leveraging technology like my Garmin watch and online tools like Training Peaks allowed me to monitor my performance and progress on metrics like heart rate, speed, time, power (watts), distance, etc. Seeing my numbers steadily improve over the years was incredibly satisfying and motivating. Maybe it was the techie-geek in me, but I loved how the metrics helped to keep me focused and positive. In fact, I used these tools to help me complete the Ironman in Kona.

In the days leading up to the Ironman World Championship, I spent a lot of time studying the Training Peaks calendar that showed all my completed workouts in green. The days of the months were full of green. I baked a mental picture of these successful training sessions into my brain. I knew the race would be extremely hard, and my mind might want to find an excuse to slow me down or stop. But if it did, I wouldn't let it. Instead, I'd pull up that mental image in my mind that proved I was ready for this challenge—I had done the work, and I was ready. Failure was not as large a presence in my imagination as success.

The third lesson I learned is to surround myself with positive people. I was fortunate to have a network of family and friends who were positive, glass-half-full type of people. And, additionally, the community of triathletes is rightly celebrated for promoting and encouraging one another.

Beyond my local social circles, I was also comfortable using the internet to reach out and connect with other athletes from around the world. I was never really worried about introducing myself and asking for advice. The worst that could happen is someone wouldn't reply, or they'd tell me they couldn't help. Fortunately, that never did happen, even when I was asking advice from athletes I'd be competing against.

Going into Kona, I was armed with no less than eight detailed race reports and recommendations from athletes who had done this race before. This included both able-bodied athletes and those with disabilities from all over the world.

Since that time, I've been the one who is asked to provide advice and suggestions, and I've always done it with enthusiasm. Sharing what I've learned makes me feel good. I get to relive my races while helping someone achieve their dreams.

On the topic of surrounding yourself with great people, I had no problem being selective. For me, even if it was a family member, if they didn't think that I could (or should) accomplish a goal that I had set for myself, I'd purposely spend less time with or around them. I knew my community was key to my success, so I was sure to be the one who defined it and kept it positive.

And the last lesson I've learned, or maybe it was something I simply reconfirmed, was to work your ass off if you want to achieve something significant. Hard work has been the key to all that I've accomplished in life—from growing up working with my dad and brother in construction to my education, career, marriage, rehab or training—and without a solid and smart work ethic, I never would have been as successful as I've been.

The great thing about this lesson is that I don't think working hard is simply an innate gift that I was blessed with. Yes, I had incredible role models in my mom and dad, but it was a conscious decision, too. I've learned to enjoy working hard because it never fails me. I made it part of my identity that brings me pride. But this isn't unique to me or a few. Working hard is available to everyone.

Focusing on what I can do, setting achievable goals, surrounding myself with positive people, and working my ass off were the four keys to my recovery, and my life in general. Focusing on these key lessons learned helped me accomplish the seemingly impossible and facilitated rebuilding my life after so much had been taken away.

With the Ironman behind me and finally feeling like I was recovered, in 2018, I was ready to start the process all over again.

Chapter 12

Not Again

"It's not what happens to you, but how you react that matters."
– Epictetus

I tried to embody this idea when I broke my back. I was terribly unlucky to lose the use of my lower body and suffer so many of the complications that accompany a catastrophic spinal cord injury. But I could still move my arms, and I could still dream. I would use what I had to prove to myself and the world that anything was possible.

The Ironman was the hardest thing I'd done in my life. At some level, I can't even believe it happened. This epic race allowed me to stretch myself beyond the confines of what I knew was possible, and I'll always be grateful for the opportunity and the outcome. I might always suffer from pain in some form, but I've experienced how crucial it is to keep my mind open and to lean into the possibilities of an amazing life. It's the only way to live, regardless of the challenges I might have.

I was determined to accomplish things that would make my girls proud, and I think I succeeded. I wanted to end this book here, as it really is the best part of my story, and it's not even about me. Looking at life post-Kona, I realized that the entire experience has helped define for both my daughters what is possible when you stretch yourself and push your limits. In many ways, the Ironman gave me the opportunity to prove to my children that anything is possible.

What's Next

Following the World Championships, I started seeing this attitude and confidence in Chloe and Zara. Strong, focused, hardworking, conscientious, and committed. Seeing these traits in your children is wonderful for a parent. At the time of writing this book, Chloe was excelling in ballet and preparing to graduate high school from Canada's National Ballet School, and Zara was accomplishing great things academically and as an up-and-coming equestrian. In 2019, Zara was accepted as the youngest member of the Ontario Equestrian's Development team, called GRIT. Both my girls were unstoppable.

Remember those questions I asked you to think about before I started my story: what's the worst thing in life that could possibly happen to you, and the hardest thing you're dealing with today?

Before my accident, breaking my back would have been on the shortlist of the worst possible things that could happen to me. But it did. And I had to respond. I was determined to get my life back and be the best husband, dad, and person I could be. With two little girls at home watching me, I had the best reason to get out of bed and try my hardest. My daughters didn't care that I could no longer walk, and that was perfect.

With the help of Sabrina, Chloe, and Zara, I found a way to live again, and together, we made a really good life for our family. Life was great. Until, out of nowhere, on Monday, September 21st, 2020, the truly worst thing in life that could possibly happen, did. Zara went for a ride with her mom and was involved in an accident with her horse. And she never came home. My little girl died. She was only 14 years old.

It had been a typical Monday afternoon for all of us. Chloe was in residence at school, and Zara had enjoyed her second Monday of high school. Upon getting home, she and Sabrina grabbed a snack, fed the animals, and got ready to head to the barn. I was working on my computer on the couch when Zara came and gave me a kiss before heading out again. She always gave me a kiss before she left the house. And as the door was closing, she would say, "Love you." I'd respond, "Love you, too. Be careful."

With the house empty again, I headed to the basement and completed my handcycle workout on the trainer. A couple of hours later, back on the couch and having finished my dinner, my cell phone rang. It was Sabrina's phone calling me, but someone else on the other end.

"Zara's been in an accident. Come to the hospital." I asked if Zara was conscious, and she replied, "No." FUCK!

Zara and Sabrina had gone for a trail ride off the barn property and through a neighbouring farmer's field. In the past, they had enjoyed exploring the different paths surrounding the barn and would share with me what they found when they returned home. As Sabrina later explained to me, on that evening, Zara was leading and decided to go a little further when they came upon what looked like a large muddy patch with ATV tracks running towards it. Zara, being the more confident rider on the more predictable horse, started walking her horse forward over this muddy ground when all of a sudden, her horse sunk into the bog up to its withers.

There was panic as her horse went further in trying to find his footing, and they were suddenly behind some trees. Zara rolled off and found her footing and called out to Sabrina to let her know what happened. Her mom asked if she was okay, and she confirmed that she was. She then pulled out her phone from its belt holster, took a video of her horse's situation in the bog, sent it to Sabrina, and told her to call for help from the barn manager, who would know what to do. In finding her footing, Zara and her horse moved down the bog somewhat, and Sabrina could no longer see them behind the trees. She was positioning herself along the trail so that those coming from the barn could see where they were and she could wave them in. Sabrina and Zara hollered back and forth with updates. Zara said she was going to ensure her horse's head stayed above the water.

Barn staff arrived shortly but had trouble getting around to Zara in their ATVs. After checking with her on foot and with her assurances that she was okay and wanted to stay with her horse, they left her to quickly find a way to get the machines and rope to the other side of the bog. This would make it much easier to pull the horse to safety. But when they got around to Zara again, she was gone. All they could see was her hand reaching above the surface of the murky water.

Sabrina heard them screaming her name as they pulled her out and started CPR. Sabrina called 911, and someone came to get her horse so she could get to Zara on foot, climbing over a trunk of a downed tree. She sang to her as a friend continued chest compressions. She asked her to please wake up as she tried to clear her mouth of debris. She expected at any moment for Zara to start coughing up water, as it might happen in a movie. They performed CPR until the police and ambulance arrived and brought Zara to the Children's Hospital, where I met them.

I arrived in the ER and watched as a room full of doctors and nurses tried to bring our Zara back to life. Sabrina and I spoke loudly to Zara, encouraging her to come back, to fight, that we needed her, that she still had lots to do. After 30 minutes of chest compressions and injections, the lead doctor called Zara's time of death. She was gone. My baby drowned in a farmer's field.

As I write this, it's been less than a year, and we're still deep in grief. The waves of grief come and go and then come again. They take my breath away each time, and I can't see beyond them. It takes everything to keep my head above the water. And just when I think I'm fine, I'm hit by another wave, and then another. I struggle daily, often too preoccupied with my own grief to effectively comfort Chloe and Sabrina. This loss is immeasurable, the weight unbearable.

When I think about the challenge of recovering from breaking my back, that was easy compared to learning to live without our baby girl. My SCI impacted me the most, and I could put all my energy into fixing it, fixing me, fixing our family. But this is so much harder. There's nothing I can do to fix this. There's no bringing Zara back. We're all so crushed and damaged by her loss. And the gaps between what we know.

We know we need to move forward, to find a way. Even if it's slowly. Life is precious, and we need to live, somehow. For the first six months, I didn't think I could ever speak publicly again. But slowly, I started asking myself, "What would Zara do?" She was so kind and giving and selfless. She'd want to help others. She gave up her life saving her horse. Rescuers were able to pull her horse out of the bog, and he made a full recovery. Just as Zara would have hoped. I wondered, *Do I still have a story to share, and am I strong enough to share it?*

What about the four key lessons I learned from my first recovery? Do they still apply? Do they work when the worst thing you could imagine happening actually does?

The first key was focusing on what I had, not on what I'd lost. Today, I must focus on who I still have. Not on losing Zara. Chloe and Sabrina still need me, and I need to help them and my extended family and friends with any challenges they're working on. I need to stick around to do what I can.

The second key focused on goals. Zara accomplished so much in her short 14 years. The last night I kissed her before going to bed, she was at the dining room table sewing a new Covid mask with her Nani's sewing machine. She had figured out how to operate it all on her own. She would have wanted me to keep moving forward.

In preparing myself for my first meeting with my psychologist, I wrote down my goals for the 12 months following Zara's death. It was simple, and singular: to survive. I figured if I could get through the first year in one piece and not damage or hurt anyone I love or blow up my marriage, that would be a huge accomplishment. Anything else I do would be a bonus.

The third key to my recovery was surrounding myself with good people. In trying to work through the loss of my little girl, I needed loved ones closer than ever. But because of the Covid-19 pandemic, almost everyone was being forced to stay away. This only made grieving and mourning harder. Fortunately, a few key people disregarded the rules and visited our bubble and made life more bearable. Many others found new ways to reach out, like texting a heart emoji when they were thinking of us. The virtual support was nowhere near as good as a hug, but it helped. And we were grateful for the kind thoughts, support, and love being sent our way.

The last key to my recovery was working my ass off. Looking back to 1996, when Sabrina and I got married, we worked hard to build a wonderful life for our family over our first 12 years together. In 2008, everything changed that day in the forest. Forced to learn how to live again, we did. By 2020, after another 12 years, all of us were hitting our strides—life was really good, and we were grateful.

Then, the unthinkable happened. Zara died, and we've been forced to start over—again. But this time, it's without one of the key players who made the first recovery possible; she was young, but she was a cornerstone of our family. Life just became exponentially harder, again.

Finishing this book would have been hard enough when life was moving smoothly and our family was whole. Reliving the grief that resulted from my SCI was difficult on its own, especially when traumatic memories intensified the burning neuropathic pain that I felt each day. I don't think anyone would expect sharing a story to be an emotionally and physically painful thing to do. But for me, many times during this process, it was. Then, adding the raw and seemingly bottomless grief that came from losing my daughter, Zara, to all my other challenges, completing the book became a goal even more difficult than any race I'd ever completed in my life. To find the strength required to carry on will take everything I have.

After completing the Ironman, I felt I had a neat and tidy end to my story that I could feel really good about sharing. I lost that. Losing Zara forced me to realize that my story hadn't ended. Those were just chapters. Life is not a novel with a clear, linear plot. It is continually being written, extending beyond the happy ending that may be contained within the tidy covers of a book.

Chapter 13
Today

Loss in life accumulates. Many days require all my strength and fortitude to keep my mind from being consumed with worry. At some point, will all that I've lost pile too high to see beyond, to move beyond? Even though I can call myself an Ironman, that doesn't change the fact that I still wish I could walk, dance with my girls, ride my motorbikes, and so on and so on. The importance of the things I've lost hasn't diminished because I've been able to complete one of the world's toughest endurance races. Rather, with the right perspective, goals, support, and work ethic, I've been able to accomplish significant things despite my challenges and loss. That's all I know.

In my home, I have a large photo of the moment I crossed the finish line in Kona. I've even used it for the cover of this book. I love it. It captures the suffering, excitement, celebration, and achievement that is Ironman. That was how I wanted this book to conclude. Unfortunately, now it can't.

My story has changed, and now there is no ending that I can share with you. It's as though I crossed the finish line of what was supposed to be the hardest race of my life, only to be told to get back on the racecourse and just keep doing laps. This time there won't be a finish line nor a medal waiting for me. And even though I know this, I must still somehow find the strength and courage to keep going. To dig deeper than I ever have. To withstand more pain than I ever have.

To convince myself I can survive and trust that in time, someday, somehow, I might find true happiness again, even though I'll never be whole.

Learning to live without Zara will be my life's greatest challenge. I'll strive to do my best. I must. And the next time I get to one of life's hills that seems impossible to climb, I know both of my girls will be there to cheer me up it. Chloe will be beside me, and up in heaven, Zara will be clanging her cowbell, chanting, "GO, DADDY, GO!"

Acknowledgements

I've often felt that one of the best parts of my story is how the world responded to support me, my girls, and my dreams after my accident. Whenever I shared my desire to accomplish something, and people saw me working hard to achieve it, support came from every direction. Family, friends, friends of friends and even strangers helped me. In a world where so much negativity fills the front pages and main stories of news outlets every day, it's heartwarming to see and experience firsthand the kindness of so many.

It's impossible to thank everyone who has supported me, especially when a large portion of you have been silent in the wings. But even if you've just had a kind thought about me and my girls at some point, thank you.

It would be equally impossible not to call out those who have been instrumental in my recovery as well. All the friends and family referenced in the book, please know how much you mean to me and how thankful I am. If you found yourself referred to as my "friends" in some of the passages, this was done for privacy and brevity. I'd love to have gone into depth describing so many of my cherished relationships, but the space to do this here wasn't available. For the sake of privacy or anonymity, some of the names have been changed.

To my siblings, Doralyn, Rick, and Jim, thank you for always being there for me. So much between us goes unsaid, but the love runs deep. To my mom and my dad (in heaven), thank you for teaching me kindness, thoughtfulness, and a strong work ethic. I'm trying to live up to your example. Amir and Naser, thank you. Michael and Arlen, thank you. To Sunil, Jimmer, James, Rich,

Fernando and Cheryl, you've been instrumental in my recovery and the completion of and decision to share this book, and I can't thank you enough. Though I will continue to try whenever we're together.

And of course, my deepest gratitude and love to my girls... Sabrina, Chloe, and Zara. You are my sunshine.

To learn more about Robert and Zara, you're welcome to visit:

Robert's Website: www.RockTheChair.com

Zara's Website: www.ZaraBuren.ca

Zara Buren Memorial Foundation
https://www.theocf.org/funds/zara-buren-memorial-foundation/

Made in the USA
Monee, IL
15 October 2021